I GOT PREGNANT, YOU CAN TOO!
How Healing Yourself Physically, Mentally
and Spiritually Leads to Fertility

I GOT PREGNANT, YOU CAN TOO!

How Healing Yourself Physically, Mentally and Spiritually Leads to Fertility

Underwood Books
Grass Valley, California
1998

I GOT PREGNANT, YOU CAN TOO!
ISBN 1-887424-38-5 (trade paper)

An UnderwoodBooks title by arrangement with the author. No part of this book may be reproduced in any form or by any electronic or mechanical means including information storage and retrieval systems without explicit permission from the author or the author's agent, except by a reviewer who may quote brief passages. For information address the publisher: Underwood Books, PO Box 1609, Grass Valley, California 95945.

Copyright © 1998 by Katie Boland
Distributed by Publisher's Group West
Manufactured in the United States of America
Cover design by Nora Wertz/Nora Wertz Design

10 9 8 7 6 5 4 3 2 1
First Edition

The ideas in this book are based on the author's personal experience and as such are not to be considered medical advice. This book is not intended as a substitute for medical treatment and the various medications described herein can only be prescribed by a physician. The reader should consult a qualified health care professional in matters relating to health and particularly with respect to any symptoms which may require diagnosis or medical attention.

Library of Congress Cataloging-in-Publication Data:

Boland, Katie.
I got pregnant, you can too! : how healing yourself physically, mentally, and spiritually leads to fertility / Katie Boland.
    p.   cm.
ISBN 1-887424-38-5
1. Infertility, Female--Popular works. 2. Infertility, Female--Alternative treatment. 3. Stress relaxation. I. Title.
RG201.B556 1998
618. 1'78--dc21   98-9477
                                                                          CIP

For My Precious Mimi
&
My Beloved Robert

FOREWORD

As a perinatologist whose practice is dedicated to the management of high risk pregnancies, I have, over the last few years, seen an increasing number of patients who required treatment by an infertility specialist to become pregnant. This is primarily due to two factors. First, infertility specialists are becoming better at what they do. Second, patients with underlying medical problems or other high risk factors, (such as age), which previously excluded them from conceiving or carrying a pregnancy, can now conceive with the help of an infertility specialist and successfully carry a pregnancy with the help of a knowledgeable obstetrician.

Katie Boland is one of those special patients you meet for the first time and know immediately that despite the odds, she would succeed. Her journey began with physicians telling her that she would never get pregnant, and ended with a beautiful daughter. In these pages, Katie describes how she not only survived, but took control of her mental and physical health to overcome infertility. Katie presents the techniques she utilized to maintain a positive outlook, reduce stress, and enhance her diet during her infertility experience and pregnancy.

In addition to reporting her own personal story, Katie recounts the cases of other infertility patients whose individual determination enabled them to triumph over medical uncertainty. She also interviewed numerous physicians, and other health professionals. The author has interwoven her knowledge and advice into this practical guide on how to get pregnant against all odds.

Dr. Khalil Tabsh
Los Angeles, CA

Khalil Tabsh, M.D., is a Clinical Professor, Department of Obstetrics and Gynecology, UCLA School of Medicine

ACKNOWLEDGEMENTS

This book would not have been born without the "mid-wives," to whom I am deeply and eternally grateful.

To my agent and steadfast friend, Anne Sellaro, for your conviction, your vision, your shoulder, your ear, and your voice.

To my publisher, Tim Underwood, for jumping off a cliff with me and making my dream come true.

To my editor, Kyle Roderick, for your brilliance, which is sprinkled like a fine mist over these pages.

To my cover photographer, Linda Gorgason, for your multi-purpose magic wand.

To my therapist, Lynn Ianni, for lifting me when I lay flattened and for breathing new life into me.

To Susan Hodder, for your heart, your clarity and never letting go of my hand and for baby Reed.

To Lorna Doctorow, for your heroism and for always lighting my way.

To Susan Proffitt, Lynn Beekler and Nanci Cone for your courage and your inspiration.

To Lynda Malerstein, for your bountiful chest and tender mothering.

To Mirna and Alvaro Rodas, for always being my family.

To Theodore S. Field, Jr., for your direction and your passion.

To Michele Singer Reiner and Sally Willcox for your early faith.

To Aurora and Neil Pennella, for finding me and teaching me to believe in miracles.

To Yoshi and Jim Gall, for your wisdom and guidance.

To Nina Leif for your generosity and support.

To my core group of women near and far: Carol Walkup, Sherry Trent, Ruthie Larsen, Kendall Hailey, Luanna Anders, Candy D'Amato, Toni Spencer, Julie Liefermann, Chellie Campbell, Sue Mullen, Margaret Perez, Brooke Briche, Pamela Zacha, Liz Skrodelis, Nancy Widmann and honorary girlfriend Stuart Crowner, for being my cheerleaders, my readers and my reality checkers.

To my mother and dad, Teresa and Bob Boland, who were also my readers, for your love, friendship and encouragement.

To my fellow school moms: Suzanne Dvells, Anahit Hataman, Eileen Shaw, Alena Stewart, Cindy Wayne and Barbara Weller for your pinch hitting and your many kindnesses.

To my amazing physicians, past and present: Khalil Tabsh, M.D., Ingrid Rodi, M.D., Ellen Blanton, M.D., Allan Metzger, M.D., Barbara Crandall, M.D., Mitchell Karlan, M.D., Almaia Jajour, M.D., Vera Cecilio, M.D., Alan Mandelberg, M.D., Douglas Morrow, M.D. and Edwin Jacobs, M.D., Nancy Therous, R.N., Ph.D., Michelle Fox, M.S. and Terry Bechtel, P.T., O.C.S., M.T.C., for orchestrating my many resurrections.

To my masterful, current UCLA team: Ken Kalunian, M.D., Jennifer and David Grossman, both M.D.'s, and Laurie Gregg, M.D. for your loving care.

And to my former husband and father of my child, Jimmy, for your enduring love, your extraordinary sperm count and your utter devotion to our daughter.

TABLE OF CONTENTS

INTRODUCTION

In an NPR broadcast in February 1997, demographers revealed that there has been a thirty percent drop in the birth rate due to fertility problems. Instead of tripling by the year 2200 as was expected, the population rate will not even double because of infertility.

In 1992, according to the American Society for Reproductive Medicine, 5.1 million women spent almost two billion dollars trying to conceive. By 1995, the National Survey of Family Growth, conducted by the National Center for Health Statistics, found 6.2 million women reporting impaired fertility, with about forty-four percent of them seeking medical treatment.

One year later, in 1996, the number of women coping with infertility had climbed to 7.5 million, according to Joan Borysenko, Ph.D., in her book *A Woman's Book of Life* (Riverhead Books, 1996). That's almost a fifty percent increase in four years!

Even the best fertility clinics and practices in the country can boast no more than a twenty-five percent live birth success rate, which means three quarters of all women who walk through their doors do not conceive. Clearly modern medicine doesn't have all the answers.

If the medical doctors are not going to get you pregnant, isn't it time you tried something else?

This book is a comprehensive guide to everything you can do to get pregnant, besides going to doctors. Most infertile couples are unaware of alternative solutions because they don't typically view themselves as "ill," so they've never had to search for a "cure." Because I was diagnosed with a baffling chronic illness, I was forced to look beyond traditional medicine. I also learned that the power of "mind over matter" truly exists and that emotional shifts could bring about physical changes. Once empowered with an arsenal of new weapons that had significantly improved my health, I attacked my infertility.

Everyone knows that infertility causes stress, but I also believe and found research to support that stress causes infertility. For the last five years, Harvard psychologist Alice D. Domar, Ph.D., has been conducting the first ever, controlled clinical trial of mind/body medicine for infertility. Within six months of completing her ten week program, forty-two percent of the first 284 women became pregnant! Women who had been infertile, on average, for three years. Dr. Domar is proving that by learning relaxation techniques and focusing on self-care, you can eliminate the stress that is keeping you infertile.

This book is packed with ways for you to de-stress and promote your own fertility. It presents an array of healing practioners and their techniques. It is filled with tools to help you help yourself and to help your baby come to you. And this book can help you increase your chances of success at the doctors' office.

I will also take you on my journey. The idea for this book was born shortly after my daughter was. As I held her close in those first few days, I knew I had to help other women know this joy. I knew I had to help other babies find their mothers.

I recently heard Yale cancer surgeon and mind/body pioneer, Dr. Bernie Siegel, give a speech, and he said that enlightenment usually comes from a major loss or a life-threatening illness. Infertility brings a major loss each month and many people feel they are dying inside as their infertility drags on. I realized that couples who are trying to conceive have a unique opportunity for enlightenment. Siegel also said, "Pain is great fertilizer. Use it."

I have walked in your shoes. I have ridden the roller coaster. I overcame anatomical infertility, a chronic illness, genetic problems and a family death. I had no family support, a troubled marriage and a harrowing pregnancy. And yet, I got my girl.

This book is about hope. It's not about giving up; it's about letting go. It's not only about getting your baby; it's also about getting your life back. I know because it happened to me. I nearly lost my myself before I found my child. Before I could find her, I had to find me. If I could do it, so can you. And I can show you how.

Katie Boland
December 1997
Los Angeles, CA

CHAPTER I

MY TRAIPSE THROUGH THE MAZE

"You can't be brave if you've only had wonderful things happen to you."
—Mary Tyler Moore

—May 12, 1989....Northridge Hospital, Northridge, CA....9:20 p.m.

As I lay on the delivery room table clutching my husband Jim's hand, I heard my baby daughter's first cries. It was the most profound moment of my life. My child was here at last.

Jim looked at me incredulously and said, "My God, we made a baby." I told him I loved him with all my heart.

Maria Rose, aka Mimi, weighed in at five pounds eight ounces, an exceptionally high birthweight in light of her six-week prematurity. Once she was swaddled and placed in her Daddy's arms, he brought her to me while the doctor mended the incision from my C-section. My joy knew no bounds.

"Who does she look like?" Jim asked.

Her tiny, squinched-up face looked exactly like his and so did her headful of black ringlets. I held her wondrously soft cheek against mine. "Hi, Mimi. It's Mommie. Happy Birthday, Angel Baby. I love you forever." I gave her a quick, teary kiss before Jim whisked her off to the Neonatal Intensive Care Unit for observation.

"Talk to her," I urged him.

I could hear Jim cooing to Mimi as he hurried down the hall. Less than ten minutes after her birth, she was gone, and I felt the first lurch of maternal separation anxiety.

As my doctor, the supremely gifted Dr. Khalil Tabsh, who was then Obstetrics Chief at UCLA, stapled me shut, he marveled "I don't know how you ever got pregnant! Your tubes look completely blocked!"

I felt omnipotent. He knew that I felt I'd received divine assistance in getting pregnant and staying pregnant and he'd always been respectful of my process. But now he could actually see the barriers I had overcome.

"At best, this should have been an ectopic pregnancy," he continued. "I thought I was going to have to do a hysterectomy to remove the placenta. You've got massive scar tissue."

I felt high on the realization that I had accomplished a supernatural feat. I had been an obstetrical no-go, diagnosed with blocked tubes stemming from an undetected chlamydia infection ten years earlier. I had endured multiple surgeries and drugs, spanning three years of infertility. I had suffered the onset of a chronic illness and the death of my baby brother. Doctors had repeatedly insisted that I would never get pregnant, and that I could die if I did.

I was beaming as if I'd swallowed the sun.

Tabsh grinned in amazement. Then he issued a proclamation: "This baby is a miracle!"

I gestured to the heavens and whispered, "I had lots of help."

I had also helped myself. And yes, she was a miracle.

****

December 24, 1978....Fairfax Hospital, Fairfax, VA....Evening

I was fresh from my first divorce, alone, and very sick. Being single brought new freedoms and new opportunities for sexually transmitted diseases. I had a new infectious strain that was not responding to traditional antibiotics. A dark figure hesitated in the doorway of the hospital room. Something about him looked familiar. It was the Roman collar.

He patted my hand. "Allow me to give you the Last Rites, my child."

"I'm not going to die!" I wailed and pulled my hand away from his. He smiled patiently.

"Would you like Communion?"

"I'm a lapsed Catholic," I shuddered.

"Perhaps I could hear your confession."

"Perhaps you could leave."

He blessed me and shuffled out.

I hugged myself tightly. I knew I would survive. I was only twenty-six years old. My life had been a succession of false starts. I felt like it hadn't quite caught fire yet.

My parents pinched pennies to educate my five younger brothers so one day they could support their own families. "You can marry a college graduate, Katie. We have to send the boys," explained Mom, when no school money was forthcoming. I paid my own way through three years, then dropped out to marry my college man at age twenty-one. I then supported him through his senior year and watched the rest of my class graduate without me. Not getting my degree is one of the very few regrets I still carry with me. And I remind myself as I write this that it's never too late.

My first husband and I were playmates more than partners. He was a struggling musician and I was working as a sales rep for a big cosmetic company, covering their Baltimore/Washington D.C. territory. I loved my job even though I knew it wasn't my life's work. I had a company car, an expense account and all the make-up I could fit into our apartment; but I soon grew tired of being the responsible partner.

Our marriage lacked the structural integrity that might

have sustained us through stormy weather. Four years from my wedding day, I was officially single again.

Now hospitalized after a year of loose singlehood, I was fighting to hang on until my gynecologist, in whom I had great faith, could save me.

I nicknamed him Dr. Columbo because of his rumpled clothes and hair. The only time he fell off his pedestal was when he installed my IUD. He wanted to wait until I was having a period. I didn't, and he only gave in after prolonged begging on my part. He should have held me off because, as it turned out, I was pregnant. I had gone off the pill after ten years to give my body a break. But I hadn't taken a break from sex. *Lesson #1: (the first of many Life Lessons I learned the hard way) Never take "time off" from the pill.*

The gentleman who was fifty percent responsible for my condition had fled upon notification. He mailed me a check which bounced, for my subsequent abortion and IUD removal.

Now I felt sure God was punishing me. *Lesson #2: Abortions don't cause fertility problems unless they're botched.*

At the hospital my family hovered around my bed with grave faces: peritonitis had set in. Dr. Columbo summoned my father into the hall, and I overheard, "We just lost a girl about her age last week with the same thing." Nearby, my funeral arrangements were being argued at top volume. My family "solved" everything with opinionated voices talking over one another. I felt very weak yet very alive as I listened to them writing me off. It's funny now; it wasn't then.

My doctor finally discovered through lab cultures that the then little-known chlamydia bacteria was the culprit. He dosed my body with different antibiotics, and two weeks later I was discharged into the waiting arms of my live-in boyfriend— whom I suspected had given me this new and exotic venereal disease. (Two years later I married him anyway. I thought I was in love; and besides, he had a Masters degree.) Please forgive me if my life sounds more than a little crazy. It was. Today, I look back on my youth and see how my romantic and marital misadventures grew out of emotional vulnerabilities and a confused identity. Like everyone else on this earth, I wanted more than anything to love and be loved. The problem was, I couldn't realize this ideal until I learned to love myself. As a result, I made a series of bad choices. No wonder I harvested serial unhappiness.

****

I was raised in a rigid, Roman Catholic home by an iron-handed FBI agent father and a homemaker mother who literally boiled our toys when they fell out of our cribs. (My mother was very devout and 'Cleanliness is next to Godliness' was her doctrine. Consequently, no one could ever describe me as being even remotely neat.) As a little girl I longed for her, but with five younger brothers, and the first four of us born within three and a half years, she was engulfed by backbreaking demands.

Every time my mother went to the hospital to have another baby, I felt abandoned and lost and crushed without her smell, her voice, her touch. My father tried to console me, to pincurl my hair, but nothing helped. I wanted my Mommy. No one recognized the depth of my distress. When Mom finally did come home, she had another needy, crying infant to take care of, and that meant even less time for me.

As a young teen, I craved my father's praise, but like many young women throughout history, I was not cherished. After being the good girl for years, teenage hormones hit and the little girl whose needs had gone unmet for so long exploded with rage against her parents. I had developed a tough crust but I still thirsted for Mom and Dad's love and approval. And they were overworked, stressed out, and ill-equipped to meet my emotional and psychological needs.

Before I signed on with Mr. Most-Likely-To-Have-Given-Me-Chlamydia with the Masters degree, my parents had badgered me relentlessly to legitimize my living situation. Desperate for their blessing, I warily married again at twenty-eight.

Shortly afterward my gynecologist gave me the bad news. "We think patients who have had chlamydia could have trouble getting pregnant." He then advised me to play it safe and stay on the pill.

(It is now common knowledge among medical professionals that undetected chlamydia is a leading cause of infertility in women. It would be years before I would know how much damage it had wreaked on my reproductive system.)

I doubted, then, whether I wanted any children. Although I lacked a master plan for my life, I vowed never to end up like my mother, struggling to raise six kids on a tight income. Then my brother Matt and his wife Janet had my niece, Alyssa, and she changed my mind. From the moment I held her, I knew I had to have my own child someday.

Truthtelling was uncommon in my second marriage and there were many questionable incidents on my Mr.'s part. It became obvious this relationship would not support a new addition. At thirty I felt much older and very disheartened. After surviving two benign breast lumpectomys and a brush with cervical pre-cancer, I quietly filed for my second divorce.

"Breast lumps are benign in ninety to ninety-five percent of cases," says Dr. Mitchell Karlan, my doctor and a leading Beverly Hills breast surgeon. He cautions that only a surgeon can determine if a lump is a cyst, which occurs fifty to eighty percent of the time and can be needle aspirated, or a nodule, which requires minor surgery.

As it happens, five percent of women each year receive an inconclusive diagnosis of their PAP smears, according to Dr. Richard Levine, vice chairman for clinical affairs of obstetrics and gynecology at Columbia-Presbyterian Medical Center, (New York *Times*, 6/22/97). They may require further testing in the form of a colposcopy and/or cone biopsy, as I did.

But the fates were working overtime and love didn't take long to find me once again. By 1983, I had my own image consulting business in D.C. That same year, I flew to New York to pitch a make-up video idea to a senior executive at a large studio. He turned out to be my future husband, Jim.

We had arranged to meet at the Parker Meridien Hotel. He hobbled in with a broken foot. I surprised him by pronouncing his name in perfect Greek. (My second husband had been Greek.) We ordered champagne. He told me my video idea wasn't bad, but wasn't viable without a big name or a million dollar budget. Then he asked me to dinner.

He hailed a cab with a crutch, which I found terribly endearing. We found an intimate restaurant (I have no memory of what I ate) where we poured out our life stories. We each knew instantly that the other was all we had ever wanted and been waiting for. We fell hard and fast.

The three qualities I find sexiest in a man are intelligence, a sense of humor and a big heart. Jim was brilliant, hilarious, fair and caring. He wooed me with fervor and charm and earnestness. I felt adored.

We had everything in common except music. He asked me if I liked Bruce Springsteen and I asked if he was the guy on "General Hospital." He took me to see the Eurythmics and I thought Annie Lennox was a man. He told me The Police were going to be at a party we were going to and I asked him why the cops were coming.

Our dating was a rush of mad parties and trips, to London, to Cannes. Three months after we met, I wrapped up my business in D.C. and moved in with him. (He had a law degree!) I found a great job as a Beauty Editor for a new women's magazine. The editor didn't ask me for writing samples and that was a good thing, because I didn't have any. I'd never been published in my life. I just knew I could do the job, and talked my way in. They weren't paying much, but it didn't matter. I loved the job and it gave me the freedom to travel with Jim.

His family was disappointed that I wasn't Greek. My conversion to the Greek Orthodox religion began when we became engaged nine months later, but his family kept their distance, which included speaking Greek in front of me. To them, I was still mostly Irish (and a little French) and Jim's siblings called me "whitebread."

I would be the first non-Greek ever to infiltrate his clan.

Because we were planning a future together, I felt compelled to outline my medical history, including the fact that my youngest brother Robert had Duchennes muscular dystrophy, which is terminal, and a form of MD passed from mothers to their male offspring.

There was a fifty-fifty chance of my being a carrier. The problem was, no carrier testing existed at the time. The best I could hope for was to get pregnant, have amniocentesis, and if it was a boy, have a second trimester abortion. Since there was also no way to test the fetus for the actual disease, I could be aborting a normal baby. Because the research was not promising, the doctors advised me against having children altogether.

I remained committed to my future goal of having my own child someday.

With wedding plans underway, I wanted more current information about my childbearing status. Through friends, I found a doctor who was supposed to be a whiz with cases like mine. I immediately nicknamed him Dr. Iceman because he was as cold and steely as his office. (He has since gone from being a sixties pioneer abortionist to a rabid Right-to-Lifer.) Dr. Iceman recommended a laparoscopy, and told me that during surgery he would shoot dye through my tubes to see if they were open. I underwent the operation (usually an out-patient procedure) and was hospitalized for four days, so the doctor "could keep an eye on me."

Dr. Iceman didn't appear until day two, however, when he

coolly informed Jim and me that my tubes were blocked. He put my chances of conception at twenty percent. Since we knew fertilization occurred in the tubes, we questioned this contradiction, but he shrugged and said "Things can change." That was it. He excused himself and I dissolved into tears. *Lesson #3: Glorified gynecologists are not fertility specialists.* Jim reassured me that he still wanted to marry me. In the back of my mind, I consoled myself with "We can always adopt" and besides, the parenting issue still seemed far away.

We had a grand Greek wedding with 250 guests and twelve attendants. (It was Jim's first time.) At the reception at Sardi's in New York, Jim's best friend made a toast that included a line from *The Godfather*, "...and may your first child be a masculine child." That spooked us both.

We honeymooned in Rome and the Greek Islands. Once home, I felt driven to begin my other journey, at last, for a child.

The only time I ever had unprotected sex, I'd gotten pregnant. Ironically, fertility ran in my family. (Despite the fact my mother wore toilet paper on her head to bed!How attractive!) The thought of throwing out the pills and jumping into bed had an illicit, adventurous quality to it. I felt reckless with abandon.

My husband was scared but I believed in priming the pump and told myself that if an "amnio" revealed a boy, "I'd just abort." I seriously doubt I could have gone through with it, judging from my first torturous experience and my relationship with my brother Robert. But I am an eternal optimist, I have the patience of a gnat, and I lived in great denial, so I dragged Jim along with me. I had no rationale for charging ahead except my deafening biological clock at age thirty-two, which of course, Jim could not hear.

Like most women of my generation, I'd postponed pregnancy for more than a decade. Now I was nuts. My previous mindset had been Avoidance and Prevention, and my body had gotten the message. I had no idea that a reversal of thinking would take so long for my body to implement.

****

As with most other life-changing decisions, women and men travel vastly different routes to arrive at the decision to become parents.

It should come as no surprise that women know exactly what they want. We've planned our weddings and named our children since we could jump rope. (As my friend's five-year-old explained, "I'm wearing lace gloves to my wedding so I won't suck my thumb.") Men of my generation were taught to get good jobs, get married, and pay for everything.

I don't know about you, but it seems to me that most women romanticize motherhood, while many men tend to be more practical. In the last thirty years, the rise in the divorce rate has created generations of people who come from fractured families and therefore have hazy ideas about what a family should be. Nationally syndicated columnist Ellen Goodman writes that only three percent of families today are nuclear, i.e. first marriage for both, dad works, and mom stays home with the kids.

Some conflict between men's and women's expectations is inherently in place. Comedian Mort Sahl explains: "Women marry men hoping they'll change. Men marry women hoping they'll never change. Both are inevitably disappointed." Such difficulties often escalate when coupled with the pressures of trying to conceive. As mutual understanding withers, each partner becomes blinded by their own wants and needs.

Jim felt very content with our lifestyle. Not me. If women on welfare and girls barely teenagers were getting pregnant, why couldn't I? So I sought out yet another "leading specialist on the cutting edge" and was referred to a guy who reminded me of a member of the Stepford clan—perfect hair, perfect teeth, perfect office, etc. After I relayed my story, he held my hands and told me in his velvet voice, "Go home and enjoy your new husband."

"But I had chlamydia," I protested.

"Just relax and give it a year."

I left the office confused.

Dr. Iceman had given me doom-and-gloom and Dr. Stepford was telling me I just needed more time. Wanting to believe the latter, (and much to Jim's relief) I stuck my head in the sand.

Soon after, I was offered a management position with a top-drawer, international cosmetic company. I loved my job at the magazine and wasn't eager to reenter the corporate world. But the salary and benefit package persuaded me to accept.

I should have heeded my intuition, for the corporate culture featured rampant sexual harassment and gender discrimination. The backbiting and infighting soured what could have been a positive and productive work experience.

"There's a reason they're paying you all that money. The job's not supposed to be easy," Jim reminded me.

I couldn't believe it was supposed to be so hard. When one of my bosses threw a legal pad at me during a meeting, I knew in my heart I was finished. My forthright nature threatened my superiors; no wonder my more pliable colleagues fared better.

I stuck it out for eighteen months until Jim received a terrific job offer in Los Angeles with another major studio. I was so excited to get out of New York I could have flown without the plane. Since I had studied in the theater and am a dreamer by nature, I formed the naive notion that here was my opportunity to make it in Hollywood. (Never mind that I hadn't played a part since college.)

We made the move and I discovered, much to my dismay, that there wasn't a burgeoning market for thirty-three-year-old actresses (I said I was twenty-seven) with no acting credits. A new friend suggested that it could be my pictures that were holding me back.

So I spent the next few months, and several hundred dollars, in search of the flawless head shot. Jim had been mostly amused by my efforts until he saw the scores of photos and the accompanying invoices. I did manage to land a small part in a Shakespeare production at the Old Globe Theater. I was the only cast member who was married and lived in a house, and I felt totally out of place. My fellow actors had a hunger and ambition that I didn't share. After a few soap auditions, I shelved acting for good. Jim asked me when I planned on getting a real job and I told him I was going back to work on resolving my fertility issues.

I loved to walk around the studio lot and scout for celebrities. Jim was appalled at my enthusiasm. When friends visited, we'd stroll the grounds, often spotting Meredith Baxter and Michael J. Fox from "Family Ties," or Shelley Long and Rhea Perlman from "Cheers." Once I sat at a table next to Jack Nicholson in the Executive Dining Room and could barely swallow. Jim threatened to bar me from the studio. I guess I was a little Lucy Ricardo in those days.

Now that we were in a house instead of an apartment, I got a puppy to mother while I waited for the real thing. So Baby Alex, a seven-week-old Weimaraner, became part of our family. We thought he was beautiful and wouldn't shed; he didn't, but he was stubborn and highly excitable.

Nothing could squelch his exuberance. After spending thousands of dollars in obedience training, I asked the vet when Alex might mellow out.

"Not until he's six or seven."

"Years?"

"If at all."

(At age nine, he finally slowed down because, sadly, his back legs started to give out.)

****

As a science, infertility is inexact. As a business, it is volatile and highly-charged. Doctors cannot explain or quantify conception. It is characterized by uncertainty and mysterious occurrences. Anything can happen, and often does.

The medical community diagnoses infertility when unprotected intercourse for six to twelve months fails to yield a pregnancy, according to Barbara Eck Menning, Founder of RESOLVE, the national infertility support group.

I define infertility as a condition that exists when you are not pregnant and you want to be.

For that period, no matter how brief, you know the feeling of being unable to reproduce on demand, of being denied something you thought you were entitled to, a reward you thought was rightfully yours.

I believe that both physical and psychological factors can impair fertility. Although the psychological ones are often overlooked, many of them, like the physical, can be corrected or improved upon once identified. I think it is a mistake to treat only the physical factors. Especially because after thirty, most couples are playing beat the clock.

"We know that fertility drops dramatically at age thirty, again at thirty-five and again at forty," states Dr. Jessica Shairer, a Los Angeles psychologist whose clients include many struggling to have a family.

After unassisted efforts to produce a pregnancy have proven fruitless, it is often the wife who initiates the formal quest.

While Jim dove into his new job, I networked enthusiastically and found a fertility clinic that had a great reputation. (It has since been repeatedly sued for malpractice.) This was a difficult step for me because I was publicly admitting that I needed more specialized care. When I made the appointment, I found the doctor required a session with both of us. This was to be Jim's first foray into the process.

The first step involves a detailed fertility evaluation.

Lesson #4: Fertility problems are not always the woman's. According to the national infertility support group RESOLVE, it is a female problem in forty percent of cases, a male problem in forty percent, a combined problem in ten percent and unexplained in ten percent. Depending on the outcome of the work-up, more tests and investigative procedures may be required.

The woman is charged with determining the timing for intercourse and calls her man to duty. Sex-on-demand runs counter to his idea of spontaneity, normally a key ingredient for his arousal. While his wife lies dreaming of babies, the future dad has to perform. If blessed with a sense of humor, most couples survive these stages with minimal anxiety and emotional pain.

At this first appointment, Jim was late and the doctor kept us waiting for half an hour. I felt extremely agitated and impatient. Although I didn't realize it at the time, I had never taken full responsibility for my physical and mental health. Naively, I just wished for this doctor to wave his wand and fix me. He was a stern, humorless man with the largest hands I had ever seen. I quaked at the thought of an internal exam. I named him Dr. Palms. He said that he would examine me, and also would need a sperm sample from Jim. While I was undressing, I glanced out the window and saw my husband buying a magazine at a newsstand across the street. I later learned that the nurse had given him a dogeared copy of *People* magazine with Brooke Shields on the cover to go along with his plastic cup.

We met back in Dr. Palms' office, and he told us that Jim had the highest sperm count he had ever seen. Apparently forty million was normal. Jim's count was 160 million! Jim started smacking his chest and expounding on his Greek heritage. Palms told us, however, that he thought my tubes were blocked and I needed tubal reconstruction surgery immediately. He opened his calendar to set a date. I felt uneasy, things seemed to be moving too fast.

I knew this man had yet to see my medical records because there wasn't time to forward them from New York before our appointment. We felt we were being pushed, so we asked more questions. He became quite annoyed, talked down to us, and explained he had to open my tubes with two procedures. The first would last about five hours, and require three weeks in the hospital and three more recuperating at home. "Like a hysterectomy," he said.

During this first operation, he would install plastic devices the size of his fist (he made a fist to demonstrate and I flinched) so that my tubes would heal properly. Then I would return to have these devices removed and be bedridden for another month. We asked if a laparoscopy wouldn't be more appropriate since my last one had been years ago, and he took this as an affront. He said we couldn't afford to wait, as things could get worse. We couldn't wait to get out of there.

As we walked to the car, Jim was basking in his new Sperm Man status and delighted that he was not part of the problem. (So was I.)

I got home and called my friend Dr. J. in Washington D.C., who is an OB/GYN. I recounted our episode and he said that he'd NEVER HEARD of this procedure. He told me to buy an ovulation prediction kit and look for somebody else.

My thirty-fourth birthday arrived and I was no farther along than I had been the year before. I didn't know it at the time, but I was following the typical pattern of ricocheting from doctor to doctor with haphazard treatments and no plan.

As the fertility quest drags on, more surgical procedures may be introduced. Women remain dogged because they are advancing their cause, while men tend to grow fearful and squeamish, especially if the scalpel is pointed at them.

"What if the guy slips?" is the universal question. One male friend described his ordeal: "They tape your dick to your stomach and xerox your balls." But with their wives' wishes firmly implanted in their hearts and minds, most husbands yield.

I finally found a team of doctors whose specialty was treating women like me of "advanced maternal age." I had to wait two months for an appointment, but I considered this a good sign. The head guy was gushy and smarmy, but I was desperate and he came highly acclaimed. I nicknamed him Dr. Casanova. He recommended a laparoscopy, which he would videotape for us.

Watching my tape made me feel very mortal. It made Jim nauseous. Dr. Casanova painstakingly took us through the probe and explained that the right tube was indeed blocked, but the left one appeared to be partially opened. The procedure also showed that I had another problem: my fimbria.

The fimbria are little fingers at the end of the tube that pluck the egg off the ovary each month and send it into the tube for fertilization. These were clubbed because of scar tissue. We had two alternatives. One was a major operation where the fimbria would be separated, and while inside, the doctor would also attempt tubal reconstruction. Or he could refer me to a laser specialist and much of this could be accomplished through another laparoscopy.

I phoned Dr. J. in Washington, D.C. and he was, in fact, doing laser surgery with great results. He and his wife said I could recuperate with them the week after surgery, until I could fly home.

There were only two facilities in D.C. that had laser equipment, and one of them was a Catholic hospital that did not permit tampering with a woman's "parts." (I guess their motto was: "If God wanted you to have children, you'd be pregnant.") I was forced to wait for an opening at the other one.

Dr. J. reviewed my videotape and Casanova's findings and noticed my pre-op tests showed unusually low blood counts. I was feeling pretty listless, but figured it was due to stress. Dr. J.

didn't normally operate under those conditions, and expressed his concern that Casanova had, but because I'd come so far, he agreed to beef me up with antibiotics and go ahead. He also suggested that I see a hematologist when I got home.

Dr. J. was only able to unclub the fimbria on the left side, but the left tube was still partially opened. He told me the operation should hold up for at least a year. He added that he'd been able to clean up a lot of my endometriosis. Dr. Casanova had never mentioned endometriosis.

Armed with Dr. J's videotape, I went back to see Dr. Casanova. He shared my optimism and sent me home to get pregnant. As I left, I almost forgot to get the name of a hematologist. I was referred to "a really great guy named Bob."

So began an emotional upheaval second-to-none. Two weeks of hope, two weeks of grief and despair. *Lesson #5: Hemorrhoid remedies shrink swelling around the eyes from crying.* Month after month Jim had to appear for his regularly scheduled performances. Women have friends on the treadmill they can confide in; men rarely share with other men, fueling their isolation. While wives feel the emptiness of not having a child, husbands feel the emptiness of not having a wife.

****

By the time I called Dr. Bob, he was on vacation for three weeks, so I was relegated to his son, who I named Dr. Boob. While Dr. Boob analyzed my lab work, I glanced at the certificates on his wall. They were earned for his work in oncology; this guy was a cancer doctor!

He pored over my test results, and unceremoniously told me that leukemia might be indicated, he wanted to do a bone marrow test, and could he do it right then?

Terrified, Jim and I agreed, and a scowling nurse led me into an exam room. While I disrobed, she explained that the procedure would involve inserting into the base of my spine a syringe that would penetrate the bone and draw marrow from its interior with no anesthesia. Dr. Boob entered the room holding the longest, thickest needle I had ever seen.

He looked very nervous and I began to cry. On his first attempt, he pierced the skin and missed the bone. On his second attempt, he hit the bone but the syringe wouldn't penetrate.

"You have hard bones," he said shakily. "You must drink a lot of milk." (Translation: This was somehow my fault.) On his third try, he made it into the bone marrow, admitting he should have used a bigger syringe. I was screaming so loudly that one nurse said I was frightening other patients. Two more held me down. When it was over, Dr. Boob said he hoped he'd gotten enough tissue for the testing. I staggered out of the office and collapsed on Jim, who looked almost as bad as I did.

I waited twenty-four hours for the results, only to be told that the sampling wasn't quite adequate, and although it didn't look too irregular, Dr. Boob told us to get another opinion. I told him to get another job, "like a coroner." I slammed down the phone, swallowed a shot of vodka and two Percodan, hoping to numb my brain as well as my aching body.

When I finally checked in with Dr. Casanova, he had the audacity to chastise me for not waiting until his buddy Bob had returned. I chose to withhold my anger. Doubts about him were becoming harder to ignore, but I couldn't bear to switch doctors again. *Lesson #6: Better to get out of the ring while you're still standing than to wait until you're beaten to a pulp.* Since it had been many months since my laser surgery and I still wasn't pregnant, he scolded me and told me I had to use my ovulation prediction kit more faithfully. (As if he had to remind me. The physician's favorite philosophy: when in doubt, blame the patient.)

During my routine exam, he detected a lump in my right breast. He recommended its prompt removal because surgery

wouldn't be an option if I became pregnant. I had the lumpectomy (my third) a week later. This, too, was benign.

Jim found the next hematologist, but I had to wait because
Dr. Boob's staff had misplaced my records. They took three
months to unearth and forward them to the new doctor. He was
gentle and deliberate and could barely conceal his horror when
I told my story. It felt good to be validated. I discussed my
deepening exhaustion and emotional debilitation. He thought I
had an immune system disorder and sent me to a rheumatologist.

I later named this new guy, who was smart and kind, Dr.
Rx because of his fondness for his prescription pad. He diagnosed me with lupus. I had never heard of it. It had nothing to
do with infertility; it was *something else*, another plunge on my
roller coaster ride.

Simply put, lupus starts with an overactive immune system. When a healthy person gets sick, her body releases cells to
fight off the infection. When the infection is brought under
control, the immune system stops producing the fighter cells.
My immune system could be activated randomly, usually by
stress, and send out fighter cells to attack healthy tissue and
organs. My body didn't know when to call off the army of
attacking cells.

"Is it fatal?" we asked.

"It can be, if major organs are involved." (Mine weren't.)

"Every ninety minutes a woman dies of lupus in this country," he droned on. I felt like a fog was descending over Jim and
me. He went on to tell us that most of its two million victims
are women. (Lupus attacks more people than muscular dystrophy, leukemia, and multiple sclerosis, and more than the *combined* total of those with Alzheimer's, Parkinson's and
Huntington's chorea.) Despite its prevalence, lupus receives
little media attention and minimal funding. The cause is unknown, there is no cure, and there's some talk it might be

hereditary. Although it is chronic, lupus can go into remission. While active, it can be controlled by medication, some with heavy-duty side effects.

I felt suffocated by this news. I had no way out. Lupus wasn't going to go away. I might have to take drugs for the rest of my life. Looking for a baby, I'd discovered I had a dangerous disease. Dr. Rx told me pregnancy was possible, but it could be risky, and prematurity was common. He cautioned that during serious lupus flare-ups, conception would be unlikely. Because I was trying to get pregnant, he wanted to monitor my condition every six weeks .

I could always find a silver lining in the darkest cloud, but I was running out of sterling. Years of testing and lack of specific solutions had worn me down. Now I faced the likelihood that the stress of infertility would trigger the lupus and prevent me from conceiving. Meanwhile, Jim's traveling was increasing and interfering with our babymaking schedule. In addition, he feared that I *would* get pregnant and then not be able to care for the baby (so did I). He also feared that our sex life and our freedom would be lost forever. He was afraid I'd get fat and stay that way (so was I). I was scared of feeling trapped and abandoned if I couldn't keep up with him. My obsession was eroding our relationship, but I dug in my heels anyway.

"What about your marriage?" friends asked.

"What about it? I want a baby."

I felt a biological need to procreate, but I also felt passionately that a child would repair, deepen and enrich our marriage.

At this point, the need for more radical treatment, i.e. fertility drugs, usually ensues. Wigged-out wives have referred to this period as hormonal hell. Husbands can be called upon to give their wives drug injections several times per month. Male psyches and stomachs were not designed for this. The roller coaster is shooting straight up and down now, with no plateaus.

When I arrived for my next appointment, Dr. Casanova had received, but (typically) not reviewed, Dr. Rx's report. This was fine with me because I didn't want to talk about lupus. I wanted to talk about getting pregnant. I had just turned thirty-five and wanted to take a more aggressive approach. I begged for fertility drugs, specifically Pergonal. He wanted to start with a milder drug, Chlomid, prescribed one month at a time, with physical exams required between menstrual periods to check for complications. Then Dr. Casanova opened my file and came unglued.

He told me I could die if I had a baby. (I thought I'd die if I didn't.) He said he'd lost two women with lupus in the delivery room during his residency. (That was thirty years ago.) He grabbed an old textbook and showed me passages that said lupus mothers were at tremendous risk. Then he fished a card out of his desk and pushed it at me. It was the name of an adoption attorney. I was stunned. My rheumatologist had been cautiously optimistic. I marched out of the office and filled my Chlomid prescription. Jim and I were spending the upcoming holidays in New York, and I arranged to see a friend's gynecologist there so I wouldn't miss a cycle.

I went to see my friend's doctor who was old and nice. He showed me pictures of his grandkids, and I called him Dr. Gramps. He said I checked out "beautifully" and gave me a refill for my prescription. I left happily to enjoy the visit with Jim's family, confident that this was my last Christmas without a baby under the tree.

Back in LA the next month, I began to experience severe pelvic pain and had to be rushed to the hospital. Dr. Gramps had made a mistake. A sonogram revealed I had cysts the size of tennis balls brewing on each ovary, an extreme complication from such a low dose of Chlomid. Dr. Casanova gave me birth control pills to shrink the cysts. Now I was going backwards.

I stayed hospitalized for almost two weeks. (Our friends

were going broke sending me flowers.) On discharge day, Dr. Casanova breezed in, poked around under my gown and invited me to a Super Bowl party the following weekend. I declined. *Lesson #7: Bare necessities to bring to the hospital: shampoo and conditioner—unless you want to spend $9.99 for a tube of Alberto VO5 from the gift shop—lip gloss and chocolate.*

Because of the cyst trauma, the lupus had begun to stir. I went to see Dr. Rx and he put me on a combination of anti-malarials, anti-inflammatories, painkillers, and something for my stomach, to control the lupus and "make me more comfortable." (Whenever I called with an ailment, his response was "Have your pharmacy call me.") Since I was on the pill, I didn't worry about complicating a pregnancy with medication.

Soon after, I received a call from Yale University, where a medical study of my family was being conducted because of my brother's MD. Robert, now twenty-three, had out-lived most patients with the disease. He was the youngest of my five brothers and I doted on him. His impending death proved a constant source of pain. We talked about it often and he always fared better than I during those conversations. How brave he was!

Yale had finally perfected the carrier testing for women and they needed more blood from Robert and me. Rob was so ill he was barely able to leave the house, but he went out in the snow for me. Two weeks later I received a letter from Uta Franke, M.D., Professor of Human Genetics and Pediatrics at Yale. She said the studies showed no Duchenne's Muscular Dystrophy gene in my blood DNA, which meant I was not a carrier. She wished me luck with my future pregnancies.

Although I was grateful for the news, I still couldn't rejoice because I wasn't pregnant yet. It seemed like everyone else was. I viewed every friend's pregnancy with a mixture of jealousy and despair.

Our marriage began to sag under all the strain. Jim retreated more and more into his work and I grew increasingly more distant as a partner and buddy. My being on the pill took the pressure off him, but I lived in a cycle of no hope for three months. I think we both feared bringing a child into a marriage that was ailing. Jim and I began regular counseling together, and with a weekly opportunity for airing, we both began to feel a little better. We sold some property in New York and I set out to find a new house in L.A. I asked every prospective seller if they had conceived children in their home. That was my one prerequisite.

At this stage of the fertility quest, money also becomes a prime factor, because remaining options such as ART (Assisted Reproductive Technologies), are exorbitantly expensive. This fact understandably frightens many husbands. They often worry that the wife may not return to work if she ever gets pregnant, and that their financial reserves will be severely depleted. Since ART success rates are so low, they logically look at the return on their investment. This sends the wife into orbit.

Before Jim and I could agree on our next course of action, I sustained another heavy blow. My family called to say that Robert had died quietly in his sleep after fifteen years of suffering and just two months after learning that I was not an MD carrier. I believed he'd hung on because he wanted me to have that knowledge and peace of mind. I was ravaged with grief. The pain came in huge waves and I felt as if I were drowning. I had desperately wanted him to see me have a child before he died.

The funeral struck me as a hideous reminder of my own emptiness, of the child who had yet to grace my life. Jim could not attend the funeral back East because we were closing on our new house. I felt inconsolable. My doctor prescribed an additional cache of drugs "to help me cope" because the lupus was flaring. I felt numb and completely alone. *Lesson #8: It's best never to wear anything to a loved one's funeral that you're not ready to ditch, because you will never want to wear it again.*

****

Looking back, I am convinced that my fear and despair literally poisoned my system and fueled both the infertility and the lupus. At the time, however, I never considered accepting any responsibility for my condition. I had followed the medical script to the letter. What else could I do?

When people told me to relax, I wanted to scream. I knew they were probably right, that I wasn't helping myself by being so obsessive and miserable. But was I hurting myself? Impeding the process? No way.

And yet, Robert's death stopped me cold. It dawned on me that I had to make some changes. For a woman whose objective was conception, I was taking an enormous amount of medication. Through my haze, I managed to realize that while I was solely focused on getting pregnant, I had let all other areas of my life go unattended. I had to let go of the idea of having a child, at least temporarily, because I had a more immediate fight on my hands: my physical and emotional well-being. I had to get out of bed. I had to get away from Dr. Casanova's lecherous eye and find a way to heal myself. And I had to win back Jim.

CHAPTER II

PSYCHED OUT

"Go for it! Take a chance. There are times you must trust that silent voice inside you. The experts don't always have the right answers. According to the laws of aerodynamics the bumble bee cannot fly. I guess no one bothered to tell the bee. Keep flying!"
—H. Jackson Brown, Jr.

My post-funeral daze was punctured by aftershocks of grief and the ringing phone. Friends called to offer condolences and I left them to the answering machine. I happened to pick up one call (thanks to call-waiting) and it was Ben, a business friend of Jim's whom I had never met. He spoke to me with compassion, but I cut him off. Nevertheless, he and his wife, Sophia, persistently called and left messages. (I know now that these two were heaven-sent; then I thought they were over-solicitous.) Jim felt embarrassed and insisted I talk to them because he had business dealings with them. I could barely believe that he was making such a request of me in my state.

When they were unable to contact me by phone, Ben and Sophia sent me some books, most notably *Anatomy of an Illness* by Norman Cousins (Bantam Books, 1985), who had cured himself of a chronic disease through laughter, love, and large doses of Vitamin C, and *Love, Medicine & Miracles* by Dr. Bernie Siegel (HarperCollins, 1990). Until Robert's death had occurred, I had never read any self-help books.

I have come to realize that most people tackling infertility do not view themselves as ill. Because they are so mired in the medical maze, they may lack exposure to alternative therapies. Although I had a healthy skepticism of alternative medicine, I was ready to explore some new directions and creating some solutions to my health problems.

****

It is accepted medical fact that we can make ourselves sick and dysfunctional. Mountains of medical research have found that the brain, when stressed from negative emotions such as fear, rage, panic and depression, produces harmful chemical changes in the body. This data led some scientists to hypothesize that perhaps the positive emotions, such as joy, hope and love could do the opposite.

In 1980, Cousins joined the Psychoneuroimmunology Task Force at UCLA which was studying how the emotions and the nervous, immune, and endocrine [glandular] systems interact. The PTF sought to prove that there is indeed a mind/body link to wellness. The amount of information they amassed repeatedly confirmed this hypothesis.

In 1978, Dr. Siegel, who teaches at Yale University, founded Ecap (Exceptional Cancer Patients), a group that facilitates personal change and self-healing with "terminal" patients who have experienced striking results. Their collective data and that of others convinced me that there was a potent connection between the mind and body.

The first research about self-healing that captivated me concerned the scientific research about placebos. A placebo is defined as a substance having no medicinal value which is given to placate patients, satisfying their psychological need for medication. Yet in study after study, when one group was given a drug and a control group was given a placebo, a significant percentage of the control group reported relief and benefit.

Sometimes they enjoyed even more benefits than the first group because they had no side effects from the actual drug.

If placebos can bring about physiological change, then what's really at work here? The mind! Cousins concludes, "The placebo is proof that there is no real separation between the mind and body." Dr. Siegel confirms "...the placebo effect—the fact that about one-fourth to one-third of patients will show improvement if they merely *believe* they are taking an effective medicine... has now been accepted as genuine by most of the (medical) profession."

These authors provided countless examples of the mind at work. I began to believe I could help myself after discovering how many others had done it. More examples of the mind/body connection began to appear in my own life.

While doing course work for her Masters, one of my dearest friends Laurel encountered a woman who suffered from a split personality. As one person, she was diabetic and required daily insulin injections. When her other personality appeared, she became physically healthy and could forego insulin for days. (An insulin-dependent diabetic can barely survive 24 hours without the drug.)

During my forth breast lumpectomy (also benign), my surgeon, Dr. Mitchell Karlan, told me about a woman who had clinically "died" during an operation he was performing. He stopped the procedure, managed to revive her, and went on to finish the surgery. When the patient awoke, she exclaimed, "I can't believe I'm here! I told my sister that I was going to die during this operation." My doctor said, "Guess what? You did!" Her body had been listening.

My psychotherapist, Lynn Ianni, Ph.D., M.F.C.C., had broken her collarbone in a car accident. Her orthopedic surgeon wanted to operate; she asked if there might be a less drastic alternative. He suggested creative visualization, because of her background in hypnosis and guided imagery with her own clients. Every day for six weeks, she envisioned her bones fusing and mending. When her cast came off, X-rays showed no evidence of her injury.

I determined that if I could work through the worst of my grief, I could then concentrate on quieting the lupus. For the first time in ages, I had a sliver of hope. *Lesson #9: There is no such thing as false hope.* That smidgen of hope is what propelled me out of bed. Without it, I'd have died under the covers. In his book *Head First* (Dutton, 1989) Norman Cousins agrees, "...hope can rekindle one's spirits, create remarkable new energies and set a stage for genuine growth."

I began to believe I could help myself. I figured that I would do the footwork and leave the results to God. He was my Last Resort. Letting go was a huge step. So was taking one day at a time.

I'm not suggesting you can overturn lifetime patterns overnight. You can take baby steps. Try not to feel overwhelmed. Everyone finds their own pace. (Mine happens to be breakneck speed.) And since I had a triple whammy to deal with, I dove in furiously and tried to race to the finish line. *Lesson #10: There is no finish line. We're all works in progress.* Even the tiniest changes will make you feel better, give you back some measure of control, and advance you closer to your goal.

I began by envisioning Robert as perfect and whole. I allowed the sadness to flow through me instead of stuffing the pain down inside me. I gave myself permission to feel my feelings. *Lesson #11: Feelings aren't right or wrong. They just are what they are.* I said good-bye to him instead of desperately trying to hold on to him. I relived standing over his open casket and looking at the boy I helped raise. I felt like my heart was being ripped from my body. We had championed and inspired each other and now he was gone. I wanted him back. But death had liberated him and brought him to a better place. So I mourned for myself, not for him.

I talked to him out loud. I actually felt nearer to him in death because I knew he could hear me all the time, whereas in life, he had lived three thousand miles away. But I still missed him terribly and longed to touch him one last time.

My firm belief that Rob and I would be reunited someday enabled me to let go and move on. I also knew that he would have wanted me to be free. And so I stopped feeling sorry for myself. I stopped expecting the sky to fall on me. I made a list of things I was grateful for. I started eating healthier foods. I took walks. I kept a journal. I stopped watching violent or sad movies and watched funny ones instead. I listened to tapes that calmed me. I tried to fill my mind with only good, positive thoughts that inspired me to keep going.

I discovered through therapy that I could choose my thoughts and that thoughts created feelings which affected my behavior. I learned to stop my negativity in the thought stage so I wouldn't feel bad emotionally or physically. For example, if I started to (a) think that I might never get well, then I'd (b) feel crummy and (c) hide under the bed covers. To prevent this scenario, I would counteract the discouraging thought immediately by telling myself that I *could* get well and that I *was* making progress in that direction. That way, I never got to the crummy phase or beyond. This exercise may feel weird, but you can spare yourself a lot of worry by consciously re-programming those tapes in your head with new, positive ones. Once you get the hang of it, it becomes a powerful tool—and an ally.

As I made these changes, I decided to stop taking all of my prescribed medication. I felt these pills were adding undue toxicity to my body. One morning, when I was feeling exceptionally determined, I flushed them down the toilet. Imagine my surprise when I realized that not only did I feel fine without all those medications coursing through my bloodstream, but my body was actually learning to "listen" to my mind. In the process, I began calming down, opening up, and loving myself and Jim with renewed heart.

I began to read all the mind/body medical books I could find and discussed them with anyone who would listen. I finally contacted Jim's friends Ben and Sophia and found them to be wellsprings of grace and love. I soaked up their wisdom and kindness. They invited me to visit a friend's home in Arizona. My two weeks there equaled a kind of spiritual boot camp. I must add here that Ben and Sophia are both attorneys and hold advanced degrees. They could never be described as flakes. They taught me that there existed a whole host of opportunities and benefits that I could pursue to mend my body, mind and spirit. (Details, strategies and techniques in Chapters IV and V.) I felt peaceful and centered for the first time in my life. I started to trust that I could get well. And I knew I was not alone. A line from "The Course in Miracles" has stayed with me since then: "When you show the slightest bit of willingness, a thousand angels will join you." I've found this applies to most anything I tackle.

Some days passed more easily than others. And recovery didn't happen instantaneously. But it astonished me how quickly things began to work. I had been stuck in the dark for so long. Little by little the sun started to come out. Then I began to *expect* sunshine. And it stayed light most of the time.

Two months later, I had tangible proof that my new formula was working. My blood tests showed no sign of lupus. The medical community called it remission. I called it a miracle.

Dr. Rx whistled the theme from "The Twilight Zone" when I left his office. I was well!

Now that I had established the mind/body link to wellness for the lupus, it was a natural step to try and apply it to the infertility. I challenged my body once again. I knew overcoming my infertility would be tricky, but fresh from my success with my illness, I felt full of hope. Enthusiasm is a great antidote for fear. Once again, I needed to start at the top and use my head first before my body would fall into line.

I had been concentrating on somehow implanting a baby into my womb through drugs and medical procedures, fixated on the lower half of my body—the "bottoms up" approach, if you will. It was time to get my mind involved, because that's where maternal yearning is born. It started with my pounding biological clock, then thoughts about what it would be like to have a baby. One day, I gave my wish a voice: "I want a baby!" Then my heart chimed in, and I began longing for a child. Finally my gut followed with a sense of knowing that having a child was something I *must* do. That's how most women arrive at the decision—they think it and feel it before they act on it.

Part of my new action plan included foregoing my traditional fertility regimen for at least a few months. This decision brought me indescribable relief and emotional freedom. I stopped obsessing. I ceased keeping track of my menstrual cycle. I stopped putting my life on hold. I started writing the screenplay I'd talked about for years. I took some quiet trips with Jim.

One excursion was a company sponsored trip to the famous La Costa Spa and Resort in Carlsbad, CA. Jim's company was picking up the tab, so I went wild. When I entered the spa, I received a checklist of all the available services such as facials, pedicures, waxing, and massages. Some I couldn't quite fathom, like herbal wraps and pore renewal, but I signed up for everything. We were there four days and I never left the spa before dark. It was my first "pampering" experience and I felt sheer bliss. Because I was feeling so relaxed and cared for, I was able to reach for Jim. With the babymaking set aside, we rediscovered each other sexually.

****

Speaking of sex, conventional research has largely ignored women in its testing and trials, particularly in the sexual arena.

In a *Glamour* article from June, 1994, entitled "Why Sex Research Ignores Women," Robin Herman writes about the mounds of research and the piles of funding devoted to male impotence, which has helped create penile injections, implants, and a vacuuming device. (We have lift-off!) Comparatively little has been invested in women's problems. After all, a woman can just lie there and still participate.

In her article, Herman also notes that lack of desire weighs in as women's number one sexual complaint. Although a drug currently exists to help increase women's desire, it has been pushed aside by the FDA as a non-priority. Claimed one unnamed FDA official quoted in the article, "If this (new drug) works, we'll have women chasing men down the halls." Other male FDA advisors expressed concern that the drug "would create nymphomania, that a woman's sexual desire could become uncontrollable." (How unfortunate that medical authorities seem to feel that unless they can find new ways to treat the male's inability to get aroused, there's no point in waking up the women.)

Women grappling with infertility (and other "women's" diseases like lupus) are largely ignored too. But I had trumped my doctors and captured their attention. By eliminating most stressors or handling them differently, I had seemingly eliminated the lupus. Now I had the nerve to think I might be able to positively affect my fertility.

I set out to see if science supported my hunches. I discovered that the pituitary, or "master gland," basically controls the release of all of the sex hormones. The pituitary's ruler is the brain's hypothalamus. All reproductive action can be traced, through different bodily systems, to this one area of the brain. And this specific area is the most heavily influenced and stimulated by the emotions.[1] If we accept that we can choose our emotions, thoughts and feelings, then hypothetically we can govern this part of the brain and its effect on our fertility. The right messages could bring the right results.

The wrong ones could bring disaster. It's well known that stress and fear cause the release of the adrenal hormones, namely adrenaline, into the body. But only recently did it become known that adrenaline short-circuits your sex-drive and impairs your fertility.[2]

This stress response can literally poison the brain. Cortisol is another adrenal hormone released under stress, which not only inhibits the production of the sex hormones, but actually corrodes the brain. If you suffer stress day after day, the long term release of cortisol will kill brain cells by the billions.[3]

Fifty years ago, the first relationship between the brain, hormones and disturbances in the menstrual cycle were being explored and considered. During WW I, "war amenorrhea" (amenorrhea occurs when menstrual periods stop completely) was attributed to nutritional factors. By WW II, scientists considered these amenorrheas to be the result of emotional factors. By the early seventies, fear of pregnancy was also acknowledged as a reason for the cessation of menses.[4]

Throughout the last two decades, research has accumulated in dribs and drabs about the relationship between stress and reproduction. Little-known studies found that negative stimuli, or stress, channeled through the hypothalamic-pituitary axis could result in irregular or nonexistent ovulation. This stress could also cause progesterone deficiencies, which interfere with the embryo's ability to implant in the uterus, and tubal spasms. Male fertility was also found to be affected. In fact, stress can reduce sperm production. For example, a series of men suffered significant decreases in their sperm counts and quality obtained at the time they were required to produce semen samples for the IVF procedure.[5]

More disturbingly, it has also been noted that in some highly-stressed women, concentrations of a particular hormone can act as a *barrier* to conception, thereby completely thwarting IVF attempts.[6] (Considering the cost of IVF, you both may want to start some deep breathing before you plunk down your money.)

More sexual dysfunctions attributable to stress include a loss of libido, premature ejaculation, impotence, and the inability to achieve orgasm. The good news is that not all couples undergo long term sexual difficulties. Apparently the optimism generated from efforts to overcome infertility can offset the negative influences initially brought on by the infertility diagnosis.[7] (More evidence of optimism winning out.)

Some researchers liken the infertility experience to that of coping with the death of a loved one or coping with the diagnosis of a chronic illness. (This is why I think I qualify as an expert, having experienced all three.) Infertility is worse, I believe because there is no resolution. Every month, I would wade through four of the five stages of grief—denial, anger, depression, and bargaining. The fifth stage, acceptance, never comes for infertile couples while they are still trying to conceive. There is only the relentless repetition of the cycle, every twenty-eight days.[8]

Depression can run so high, in fact, that the suicide rate for infertile women is double that of the rest of the female population.[9] (This is, of course, a tragic and irrevocable choice.)

I knew some would call my research thin, but even though there wasn't much available, I still felt I was on to something important. My position may have seemed controversial, but I felt my footing was sure and my reasoning solid. I discussed with my doctors my theory that stress has a direct affect on fertility, and they grudgingly agreed that I had pieced together a path, illustrated in the chart on the following page.

And then the clouds parted. I discovered Alice D. Domar, Ph.D., Program Director for the Behavioral Medicine Infertility at Beth Israel Deaconess Medical Center, a major teaching hospital of Harvard Medical School. She is also the Director of the Mind/Body Center for Women's Health at the Mind/Body

THE MIND/BODY LINK TO PREGNANCY

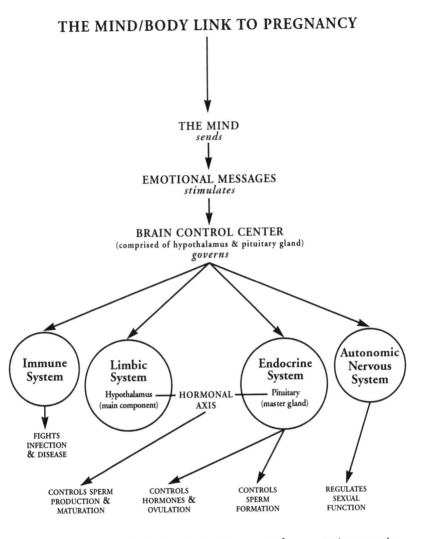

THE MIND
sends

EMOTIONAL MESSAGES
stimulates

BRAIN CONTROL CENTER
(comprised of hypothalamus & pituitary gland)
governs

Immune
System

Limbic
System

Hypothalamus
(main component) — HORMONAL
AXIS

Endocrine
System

Pituitary
(master gland)

Autonomic
Nervous
System

FIGHTS
INFECTION
& DISEASE

CONTROLS SPERM
PRODUCTION &
MATURATION

CONTROLS
HORMONES &
OVULATION

CONTROLS
SPERM
FORMATION

REGULATES
SEXUAL
FUNCTION

Medical Institute at Beth Israel. Dr. Domar is the preeminent voice and research pioneer of the mind's role in the reproductive process.

Her groundbreaking studies, begun in 1989, set out to answer the questions: Does infertility causes stress and depression? Can stress and depression cause infertility?

While I was navigating my own individual course, Dr.

Domar was investigating similar solutions on a grander scale. She spent nine years developing her methods that teach mind/body, anti-stress and healing techniques to infertile women. In 1994, she received a grant from the National Institute of Mental Health to conduct a five-year study on the effectiveness of the program.[10]

Initially fearing her program would increase participants' stress if it were viewed as just another possible route to pregnancy, Domar designed it to help participants reclaim joy and meaning in their lives. Although she suspected that conception would be a resulting benefit, she suggested that the women set this goal aside.

After two years, Domar posted some startling returns. Her work involved 284 women, who averaged three and one-half years of infertility. After completing a ten-week course in stress reduction, relaxation techniques, and group counseling, a whopping forty-two percent became pregnant within six months. thirty-six percent of the total group went on to give birth.11

The women's depression levels dropped from high to the normal range after the ten-week course. Among the women with the highest scores in clinical depression, a stunning fifty-seven percent conceived within six months. Domar concluded that depression, often caused by the chronic stress of infertility, could indeed contribute to the infertility itself. By 1998, this study will be finished. For now, we know that "mind/body medicine" alleviates the distress of infertility and promotes pregnancy.[12]

The Mind-Body Program for Infertility raised success rates for ART procedures like IVF, GIFT, etc., as well. In its premier study, thirty-seven percent of women got pregnant on their first IVF or GIFT cycle after going through the Program. Compare this to a recent trial in which twenty-nine percent of non-depressed patients got pregnant while only thirteen percent of depressed patients or patients repeating the ART procedure conceived.[13] If you want to know more, her book *Healing Mind, Healthy Woman: Using the Mind-Body Connection to Manage Stress and Control Your Life* (Henry Holt, 1996) is required reading. She has established other mind/body infertility programs in New Jersey, Ohio, Illinois and Texas. (see Resources section for more information.) Overnight weekend retreats are offered in Boston for those who don't live near a center. Domar's contribution to understanding the emotional causes of infertility is as historically important as her proposed prescriptions for its cure.

Domar's body of work confirms what I suspected all along. I couldn't prove it then. I can now. Now I can affirm with authority and certainty that *stress causes infertility. (Oh, swell. It could be in your head. It could be partly in your head. Lesson #12: IF IT IS IN YOUR HEAD, YOU CAN FIX IT.*

Couples should not feel guilty or blamed, but excited, that they can help themselves by altering their outlook and therefore their body chemistry. It can generate much hope to know that when thinking is changed, there is real physiological benefit. *Lesson #13: Don't dwell on past mistakes. Forgive yourself and forge onward armed with new energy and conviction.*

Speaking of blame, smoking, alcohol, and caffeine (Blah, blah, blah) also have negative effects on fertility. They can cause menstrual irregularities, vaginal infections and PID as well as reduced sperm counts and performance interference. (How are you not supposed to indulge when you feel crazed?)

Lesson #14: It's okay to feel lousy sometimes. Instead of suppressing my anxiety, my therapist coached me to set aside wallowing time. Then after a few hours, I would dust myself off and get on with the day.

And so I continued battling anatomical infertility, which I now know is considered harder to overcome with mind/body work than the hormonal type. But since I'd overcome the psychological consequences of a chronic illness and a family death, I felt I could actually predispose my body for pregnancy. I believed I could create the ideal conditions for conception to occur. I'd kicked the lupus. I could kick this too.

At that time, I discovered another book that profoundly affected my new thinking—*You Can Heal Your Life* by Louise Hay (Hay House, 1987). She cured herself of cancer and has helped thousands do the same. She writes that the word "incurable," which many of us find terrifying, can simply mean that a particular malady "cannot be cured by any outer means and that we must go within to find the cure." Her words spurred me on.

I know that some obstacles to fertility are purely mechanical, and therefore should be remedied with surgery. But even after corrective surgery, many couples still don't conceive. We didn't. I feel it was because, at some level, I was as stuck as I had been with the lupus. My fear and negativity sent strong messages and produced chemical changes that countered the medical treatment I was subjecting myself to. I even considered IVF at one point because Dr. Casanova had said he feared my tubes were closing up. As unhinged as I felt, I'd have done better just driving down the freeway and throwing $10,000 out the window.

****

Three months after my Arizona epiphany, another bomb dropped. Dr. J called from D.C. and asked if we wanted a baby girl that he would be delivering the following month. The mother was very young, in school and unmarried. Not yet completely free of my "quick fix" mentality, I leapt at the prospect. God had answered my prayers. Jim's standard line on adoption had always been, "I'm not raising someone else's kid." He still wasn't that keen on having his own. But after all we'd been through, I thought I could convince him.

I had to proposition him in the hospital where he was recovering from an emergency appendectomy. He was taking painkillers, but I thought this might work to my advantage. He rejected the idea immediately. He wouldn't budge. I knew I'd never get the baby without him because the mother wanted to meet both of us. If I could have surprised him, I would have. *Lesson #15: It's easier to ask forgiveness than permission.* I admit now that I was wrong.

I didn't want to forfeit my marriage. It was too late to start over with someone else. (Besides, I'd been listening for the hoof-beats most of my life. Lancelot was not coming.) The loss of this little baby girl felt almost as painful as a death in the family.

I found some comfort for my aching heart from a well-worn passage in *Words That Heal* by Douglas Bloch (Bantam Books, 1990) entitled, "Alone I Stand United."

> *You are like the man who while walking along the beach saw two sets of footprints, one his own and one belonging to God. During his lowest and saddest times, however, he saw only one set. Thinking he had been abandoned, the man cried out and asked why he had been deserted. The Infinite replied, "I would never leave you. When you saw only one set of footprints, it was then that I carried you."*
> *Alone you stand united...*

Once again, I had to piece myself together and face forward. One of my life lessons is from Larry Brown, a former running back for the Washington Redskins (my all-time favorite team in the whole world—Rob's too):

"IT'S NOT HOW MANY TIMES YOU STUMBLE AND FALL. IT'S HOW MANY TIMES YOU STUMBLE, FALL, AND GET UP."

And I always, always get up.

P.S. The unwed mother decided to keep her baby after all. Bless them both.

Chapter III

DOCTOR SHOPPING

"The thing women have got to learn is that nobody gives you power. You just take it." —Roseanne

And may I say you have one great ass," said he with the hair plugs, capped teeth and fake tan. Dr. Casanova chose to bestow this compliment while conducting yet another pelvic exam with no nurse in the room. "I bet you say that to all the girls," I shot back nervously. He propped his elbows on my spread knees and looked me in the eye. "No, I don't."

I must have radar for quacks. It started early. After my first gynecological exam at sixteen, the middle-aged doctor (then married to a former Miss Iceland) asked me out to dinner just minutes after he'd had half his arm inside me.

Then there was the gynecologist I saw drooling over a "Penthouse" centerfold when I walked by his office after my appointment.

From the psychiatrist my parents forced me to see at seventeen who came on to me, to the (alcoholic) Catholic priest and "dear friend of the family" I was then forced upon who tried to force himself on me, I have had bad luck with male caregivers.

After college, I saw a dermatologist because of a mole on my thigh. He had me remove all my clothes. "Let's have a look at you," he said as he pawed me. I felt violated, but I did nothing

41

because I was too intimidated. (I always assumed these guys knew more than me.) I'd left feeling guilty and mad at myself because I hadn't stood up to him. This pattern characterizes the way I used to handle male medical professionals and how they used to (man)handle me.

Maybe it's genetic. Shortly after she married, my mother felt embarrassed and uncomfortable about sex, as any new Catholic bride of the fifties might have. When she turned to her gynecologist for some solace and support, he told her she'd better "get with it" or she would lose her husband. And get with it she did. (After six kids I think she decided to get *off* it.)

Maybe I gravitate toward women who share my experience. When a physician friend of mine first went to Planned Parenthood as a teenager, some interns barged in once she was in the stirrups. One of them picked her name off her chart and asked, "Aren't you from that family that lives in Billingston?" She shrank. He knew her family. She was afraid he'd tell them she was there. The doctor strolled in, threw up the sheet over her splayed legs and exclaimed, "Anyone ever seen a live cervix before?" (As opposed to a what? A cadaver's?)

I think the incident that finished me off was when Dr. J. (my former friend) was accused of sexually harassing six of his patients. He told his (now former) wife, "Where am I supposed to meet women? In bars?"

And so I had an aversion to most male doctors. In recent years, however, I've met some exceptional male physicians, without whom I wouldn't be here today. That's because I became more savvy as a consumer and more assertive as a patient.

According to the American Fertility Society, *in 1992, 5.1 million women spent almost two billion dollars trying to conceive. In 1995,* the National Survey of Family Growth, conducted by the National Center for Health Statistics, found *6.2 million women reporting impaired fertility, with forty-four percent seeking medical* treatment for their condition. *By 1996, the number of women had climbed to 7.5 million,* according to Joan Borysenko, PhD., in *A Woman's Book of Life* (Riverhead Books, 1996). *That's a fifty percent increase in four years!* Clearly this epidemic is not being stemmed by traditional medical doctors, yet they're the ones who are getting the billions. (Another case made for mind-body medicine.)

It is naive to assume that all doctors have a fundamental knowledge of their fields. Doctors are not God. If they were, we'd all have children whenever we wanted them. As it is, they still can't predict when a woman will go into labor or a baby will be born. Therefore it's our job to protect ourselves while seeking out the best care possible.

We start off brimming with hope. But once settled into our consciousness, the "infertile" label induces fear. Fear fuels panic. And panic can compromise judgement. When the panic is coupled with an overzealous doctor pushing his program, escalation is inevitable. We can make fear-based decisions and borrow trouble by anticipating problems.

Cousins mentions in *Head First* that ninety percent of the doctor-related complaints he received during his tenure at UCLA were from women. He attached no significance to this, but I think it indicates that women need to raise their personal and medical consciousness and demand better treatment.

As exasperating as modern medicine can be, it has life-saving benefits to offer. Good doctors are out there. You just may have to interview a lot of frogs, and that means perfecting your screening techniques.

Strong interviewing skills rarely endear you to physicians. I and numerous friends have been told, "You ask too many questions," or "You're too upset." Well, I get upset when my questions *aren't* answered.

Another Dr. Casanova incident, of which there were many, involved a good friend who is married to a very famous film director. She was personally ejected by the great doctor himself because she became "too upset" when her labor pains started at seven months. (Bear in mind that she had been kept waiting over an hour in his reception room.) "We can't have a display in this office. You're too hysterical. Find another practice." (Dr. Casanova always prided himself on his celebrity clientele, name-dropping at the merest opportunity.) He knew full well that she'd have an impossible time finding anyone who would accept her that far along in her pregnancy. I guess that's why he has since instituted the policy that all new patients must sign forms agreeing to arbitration if there is a future dispute. (Translation: No court stuff.)

Many insurance companies mandate the forms as a condition for granting malpractice coverage. A personal injury lawyer friend assures me, however, that you can't actually waive your own rights, even if your signature is a condition for treatment.

In my experience, most doctors dislike independent-minded patients. Refusing to be led like a lamb to slaughter can make you unpopular. Dr. Siegel illustrates the point in *Peace, Love and Healing* (Harper & Row, 1989):

I'm going to draw a blood sample from Mr. Smith, and the nurse says, "That old s.o.b. won't take his clothes off, is never in his room and probably won't let you draw his blood without asking you five hundred questions while you're doing it." Whereas, if I come on the ward and say to the nurse, "Today it's Mr. Jones turn to have his blood drawn," the nurse says, "What an angel. Yesterday he had a barium enema by mistake because we have two Joneses on the floor and he never complained a minute."

Which patient do you want to be?

One night my dear friend Sherry paged her doctor, who was in a restaurant having dinner with his wife and quite tanked. He started rambling on about the Rodney King trial while she was asking to go to the hospital because she was bleeding. (She was taking drugs at home for preterm labor.) He told her to get off her feet and meet him in his office in the morning.

I insisted on accompanying her. As we were seating ourselves, her OB complained about his work load and high stress level.

"Do you want to go to the hospital?" he demanded. He was not giving her the choice as much as washing his hands of the decision. He clearly thought she was overreacting and was squirming in his seat because I was interrogating him.

I helped her decide to go to the hospital, where she was told that she could have jeopardized her pregnancy by staying home. The doctor blamed the bleeding on her emotional state and said that if she'd miscarried it would have been her own fault.

If you are feeling weak and weepy, you *must* bring a support person along with you to ask the appropriate questions and to help you remember the responses.

Even physicians suffer temporary shock and memory lapses when they become patients. I recently met a female doctor who related such a story to me. When she was told she had breast cancer four years ago, she heard almost nothing. Even though she had knowledge and familiarity with the facts when they applied to others, she couldn't process the information when it was meant for her.

Also keep in mind that some information can be omitted even by the best medical practices. When Renee, my former writing assistant, was taking fertility drugs under the care of her ace specialist and staff, she was never informed of all the side effects. Some doctors won't tell you because they don't want to lead you or plant ideas in your head. (Who says the mind isn't powerful?) Yet if things do start winging out of control, you might be told that you're imagining things. It's imperative that you learn all of the ramifications of your treatments so you don't think you're loony or dying.

Here's the scoop culled from many survivors: fertility drugs stimulate the ovaries and cause them to produce several eggs a month, thereby increasing the odds for conception. It also must be noted that they command a high price, both financially and emotionally.

More ominously, there is now some discussion among medical researchers that these drugs may be linked to ovarian cancer. Chlomid is usually the precursor to Pergonal. (Except in my friend Laurel's case. When she heard that Chlomid affected the brain, she said, "Bypass my brain. I've got enough problems.")

Chlomid thins the uterine lining, which is why it shouldn't be taken for more than six months at a time, because after that it can inhibit implantation of a fertilized egg. It can also cause hot flashes, vaginal dryness, cramping, mood swings and uncontrollable crying fits.

Perganol (derived from the urine of menopausal nuns in Italy—Really!) works directly on the ovaries and must be injected by someone else, because it's hard to self-administer. The contents of two glass vials have to be mixed and loaded into a syringe. You need to know where to stick the needle so it hurts less. The ideal shot site is that mysterious glob of flesh right around your hip line just above your buttocks. Just pinch and shoot. (Renee's husband was afraid of killing her by injecting an air bubble.) The shots hurt, the flesh hardens in this area (scar tissue) so towards the end of the drug cycle (usually ten days) the medicine can squirt back out and must be held in with a swab.

A weight gain of at least ten pounds is very common. So are night sweats and blurry vision. The shots must be given at the same time every day. (I've shot many a damp and dizzy friend because of a temporarily absent spouse.) Progesterone shots or suppositories might be added to your regimen to enhance your chances of conceiving.

Laurel summed it up: "I feel like I'm always shoving something down my throat, in my butt, or up my wazoo." Fortunately, if the drugs work for you, you will most likely get pregnant within six months. (Nothing like getting pregnant after packing on an extra ten pounds.)

Pergonal, and its sister drug, Metrodin, cost a fortune. If you live in Southern California, drugs can be obtained on a day trip to Tijuana for one-tenth of the prescription price. If you live near any borders, check this out with your doctor's nursing staff.

Fertility drugs tend to make people crazy because of their hormonal reactions to the drug, but also because expectations are elevated enormously and time limits are imposed. I know many couples who spread apart the cycles to give themselves breaks in between and reduce some of the stress.

Inseminations are often coupled with drug therapy to maximize the effects of the treatment. Hopes rise even higher. Most of my friends were convinced every month they were pregnant. Either that, or they were caught up in an anticipatory grief cycle—the foreboding feeling that doom is looming and failure is imminent. Renee wanted to know if she'd feel any different if she *were* pregnant. Would it feel like her period was coming even if it wasn't? There seemed to be no way to tell. Couldn't there be *any* delineations between pregnancy feelings and PMS symptoms? The standard answer of "wait fourteen days and we'll see" wasn't satisfactory. Those fourteen days were endless each month.

Before you decide on a doctor, consider the following cardinal rules gathered from many shop-wise customers:

1. Talk to everyone you know. Most people spend more time selecting a new car than they do selecting a doctor. This doctor-patient relationship is going to be long-term, intimate, and emotional, so invest the time before you jump in.

2. Seek referrals from satisfied patients because doctors cover for each other. (I know I saw most of Dr. Casanova's golf partners.)

3. Assume a consumer mentality. Be wary. You are the buyer. Remember, you are paying to have this done to you. If you don't think this is a business, pay attention. Fertility clinics are advertising on billboards, magazines, and on the radio. So are hospitals. They want your money. They appeal to your sense of longing. Smiling actors lure you: "Come and have your baby with us. We'll make it happen."

The American Society of Reproductive Medicine, located at 1209 Montgomery Hwy., Birmingham, AL 35216-2809, publishes a report for the public comparing success rates for clinics around the country. I strongly suggest you send for it.

4. Make sure the doctor has the letters F.A.C.O.G. after their M.D. on their door. Otherwise they are not Board Certified Infertility Specialists. This elite, nation-wide group numbers less than five hundred. To check, call the American Board of Medical Specialties (ABMS) at (800) 776-CERT from 9-6 Eastern time.

5. Schedule an hour-long first consultation. You will be charged and sometimes insurance won't cover it, but it's money well spent. How else can you know if you want to embark on a very personal journey with a stranger?

6. Ask questions with the same thoroughness you would use if you were inquiring about the options for a sick pet.

7. State any special needs you have. I have a friend who was molested, so gynecological exams are particularly painful for her. Her doctors need to know. I need to call my doctors by their first names so I don't feel one down and can feel like an equal partner. I once went to a young squirt who insisted I call him Dr. Brown. He said it was "office policy." When I explained my reasons for wanting to use his first name, he told me he'd call me anything I wanted, but he had to be Dr. Brown. I told him to forget it and walked out.

8. Let the doctor know you are shopping and see if they seem interested, not only in your business, but in you. They must be compassionate. A brilliant doctor without feelings will not allow you to feel comfortable voicing concerns. These are private matters that are difficult to discuss. Some doctors are not incompetent, just incompatible. Getting pregnant requires some hand holding. I don't know about you, but I want to feel cared for.

9. Ask what percentage of the practice comprises your age group.

10. Ask about success rates. That means live births, not total pregnancies. See if this practice is a full service operation—it should be if they are true specialists—or if they'll have to refer you out for different procedures. I would caution against this because you'll feel even more disjointed and passed around.

11. Make sure the doctors are accessible to you. How promptly will they return calls? Are there some days they're not reachable, due to surgery schedules, etc.? This will help later on if you have a burning question and can't get an answer. Ask for a back-up person.

12. Lean toward a conservative approach. Be suspicious of anyone that endorses radical procedures with dire pronouncements.

Barry Behr, M.D., director of the human embryology and andrology lab at Stanford University, stated in a March 1994 Los Angeles Times Magazine article, "Making Babies," that he fears that some clinics will accelerate in prescribing more high-tech, pricey treatment for infertile couples when lower-tech solutions might do instead. He claims that sort of practice is relatively common. "It's one of the big controversies in the field today: At what point do you resort to these aggressive, invasive procedures?" he asks.

Maybe doctors tend to suggest expensive, invasive procedures because they are hooked on the high stakes of their work. They like walking a tightrope. They are gambling with someone else's money for their own fix with very low odds for success. On the other hand, I interviewed one doctor for this book who tells prospective patients that she probably won't get them pregnant because the odds are heavily against it. Who wants to hear that?

Ann Pappert, who's working on a book called *Cruel Promises: Inside the Reproductive Industry*, commented in the same article as Behr that she feels a lot of clinics pump up the patients to ensure their return. "It's a business, and like any business, you have to keep your clients coming back."

She's not calling for a moratorium, but feels that "clinics need more supervision and safety guidelines and more deliberation when deciding who really needs high-tech treatments." She also notes that the collages of newborn which decorate clinic walls are emotionally manipulative.

Collective experience from the women I interviewed and my own hard-won lessons dictate the following course of action once you decide on a doctor:

1. If you have no reason to fear and you've never tried to get pregnant, assume you will and take a measured approach. Pace yourself emotionally. If your age is a factor, you will still benefit from a thoughtful, considered approach, rather than a frantic one. (Listen to the voice of experience. I was almost ready to steal a kid from the mall.)

2. It's best not to negotiate while flat on your back, nearly naked in a paper robe, when the doctor is looking at you from your other end. Work from a position of strength. Do your talking sitting straight in a chair, fully clothed, and look them in the eye. Bring a list of questions and WRITE DOWN the answers.

3. Ask for the names of patients you can talk to who are

already in the practice, hopefully with a medical outlook similar to yours.

4. Read their body language. Don't let them patronize you. If they're not willing to accommodate these simple requirements, what happens later when you're wearing thin?

5. Ask for any printed information so you can familiarize yourselves with process and terminology. Do your homework. Be suspicious if a doctor discourages this. Good ones don't feel threatened. You can write to RESOLVE, Inc., at 1301 Broadway, Somerville, MA 02144, for referrals and comprehensive literature.

6. Ask about the doctor's continuing education. This field is changing so rapidly that it is difficult to know all your options because they are constantly increasing. (That's the good news.) How do they learn about new technologies and more efficient procedures?

7. Ask if you can sit in on a lecture they might be giving or attending. There should be no mysteries here. You'll be surprised how much of an expert you can become without a medical degree, and how much more the doctor will respect you if you are informed. The only way to avoid feeling like you're at the doctor's mercy is to educate yourself.

8. Take control. Because if you don't, someone else will. (Everyone else will.)

9. Don't feel ashamed of your body because it's not working. Don't apologize. Remember: THIS IS NOT YOUR FAULT.

10. Don't let yourself be rushed through the office. If you can wait for them, they can answer your questions thoroughly. Your money's as good as the next patient's. If the office seems disorganized, remember that you, too, may fall between the cracks at times, and decide if this will be acceptable to you. Dr. Tabsh kept me waiting an average of two hours each visit because he was constantly being called away for emergencies. It didn't matter. He was worth it.

11. After an initial, detailed fertility work-up is completed—this is the one time where you will probably experience the conveyor belt treatment even in a good practice,—draw up an action plan with your doctor. You should be given options. They should be presented clearly and in layman's terms. The doctor's recommendations should follow. But remember, it is ultimately YOUR DECISION.

12. Ask yourself what you are willing to sacrifice. Set time limits, financial limits (only three one-hundredths of one percent of health care insurance payments in this country went to cover fertility benefits in 1994, according to the American Society for Reproductive Medicine) and reserve the right to change your mind or opt out for a month or two or three.

13. Draw an imaginary line for when you will decide enough is enough. You can move that line at any time if you decide to go from low-tech treatments to more complicated ones. (No matter what position I find myself in with anything these days, I always feel more secure if I have a contingency plan mapped out.) Take into account your age, money, travel schedules, work pressures, time of year and personality. (Do this while you still have one that's recognizable and somewhat representative of the old you.)

14. Propose a contract that both parties can sign. Birth contracts—an agreement between the couple and their doctor that states what elements they want for delivery, what medical interventions are acceptable, etc.—are becoming more widespread. Why not for fertility treatments? It's simply putting your plan on paper.

15. Don't settle for seeing only a nurse practitioner on subsequent visits. Insist on time with the doctor, even if it's only for a few minutes after each appointment, so you feel connected. If that won't work, schedule bi-monthly conferences with your doctor for ten-fifteen minutes to review progress and

next steps. Make sure you are not charged extra for these. Most people feel much calmer if they have a plan. It doesn't have to be ironclad, but should be a grid to follow and should be revised every six months (three months if you're in the drugged phase of treatment).

If you are not forthright with your doctor or an active participant in the decision making, you'll end up feeling angry and resentful if their prescribed treatments don't work. These bad feelings could negatively affect the outcome of a procedure. You don't have to waste time being mad or staying stuck. State what you want and be straightforward about how you think and feel. That's the only way to get your needs met and feel in control.

If you find you've made a poor choice, find someone else. Time and money are very precious. Don't worry about hurting the doctor's feelings, worry about taking care of yourself. Besides, you don't have to confront your former doctor. Signing a standard document authorizing the release of your records will provide the new doctor with access to them.

Here's my favorite bumper sticker:

IF YOU'RE HEADED IN THE WRONG DIRECTION, GOD ALLOWS U-TURNS...

—Jackson Brown, Jr.

I have slogged through my share of so-called experts, and even though I got angry and crazed, I persevered. So can you.

I want a doctor to give me hope. I want statistics, but I want hope too. When people have hope, they feel better, and when they feel better, they have a better chance of having other things work. I want to know that the doctor is sharing responsibility equally with me and is honest about outcomes. I won't blame them as long as they don't blame me. But they must promise to tell me the truth. I don't want to hear or read about a test and not know if I've had it and wonder if I should have or why I haven't. People tend to either deliver themselves into their doctor's hands or micromanage the process. Somewhere in the middle will keep you saner, but don't let anyone tell you you're a pain in the ass. Remember the enema!

It occurred to me that it is neither fair nor wise to entrust a physician with your entire body, mind and hope for the future. I finally learned that I was not powerless, I was not alone and that I could make a difference. I learned that I did not have to perceive myself as a victim and that I could participate in and promote my own recovery and success.

You need doctors but you also need yourself. I have accepted fifty percent responsibility for my health. My body may not always be in great working order, but my mind usually is. I am in partnership with my doctors and our mutual goal is my wellness. It's a team effort. We respect each other.

A story appeared in the *Los Angeles Times* in March 1994, written by Beverly Beyette, about the January 1994 Northridge earthquake. The author tells of a woman who was scheduled for an in-vitro fertilization procedure just hours after the disaster hit. Dr. Richard Marrs, who should be heralded for his heroics, slipped past security guards and entered his lab in the Santa Monica Medical Center. The lab was upended, but he found his patient's petri dish and five of the embryos looked viable.

He loaded them into a catheter and instructed his office to tell the woman to meet him there. He wrapped the catheter in a towel and sprinted across the street where he found the couple. A powerful aftershock hit as they were waiting for an embryo to line up with her uterine wall. Two weeks later, pregnancy was confirmed.

All of us are capable of superhuman efforts in extraordinary circumstances. But most of the time, doctors are only human. We need to remove them from their pedestals and lessen our dependence on them. Sometimes we know what's best, and that's why we deserve fifty percent of the vote. Seize it. A bad doctor won't give it to you but a good one will welcome the challenge. That's how you can tell them apart.

CHAPTER IV

GETTING PHYSICAL

"One out of four people in this country is mentally imbalanced. Think of your three closest friends—and if they seem okay, then you're the one." —Ann Landers

Before you subject yourself to any more infertility procedures, you should consider antibiotic therapy. I only discovered this course of action while researching this book, but it may save you years of anguish and thousands of dollars. The proponent of the theory is Dr. Attila Toth, a Pathologist and OB/GYN at New York Hospital and Associate Professor of Obstetrics and Gynecology at Cornell Medical College. When I finished his book *The Fertility Solution* (Atlantic Monthly Press, 1991), to which I was glued for two days, I wanted to scream from my rooftop. During my own trek and in listening to the tales of others, I had never heard of this approach and it makes so much sense. I only wish I'd found him sooner.

His premise is simple. He is convinced that the fundamental cause of at least half of all infertility is common bacterial infections. He believes that a high percentage of these cases can be easily and safely reversed with the proper combination and dosage of antibiotics. And his remarkable results prove it.

Toth began his pioneering work by asking "Why has the infertility rate continued to trend upward in the years since

1970?" He believes it's because American men and women have become more sexually active with a greater number of sexual partners, which has fueled the spread of STDs (sexual transmitted diseases), particularly chlamydia and countless other bacteria. Many of these thrive unchecked in the victim's reproductive system because they are asymptomatic until the victim or victim's partner fails to produce a child.

Another reason for the upward trend is, logically, that women are putting off childbearing until their thirties and forties, which allows STDs more time to weaken their reproductive powers. Toth says that when many doctors diagnose infertility problems as premature menopause, he has been able to reverse the damage and restore the victim's fertility with antibiotic therapy.

He also maintains that certain bacteria in human semen can adversely affect the shape and motility of sperm, rendering a man "infertile." Antibiotic therapy can cure and restore the sperm to its well-functioning form.

The study that vaulted Toth into the *New England Journal of Medicine* and was reported in the *New York Times* consisted of 161 couples. All of them took 100 milligrams of doxycycline twice a day for four weeks. In 129 cases (eighty percent), the husbands' bacterial infection was successfully eradicated. Seventy-seven couples (sixty percent of the 129) went on to successful pregnancies. For the remaining thirty-two couples in the study whose infections were not eradicated by antibiotics (as evidenced in post-study semen cultures), only two (five percent) became pregnant.

Most women conceive between three to six months after completing his prescribed course. Many who find Toth are at the ends of their ropes. The point is, he should be the *first* stop.

Toth tells of one couple who had tried for three years to get pregnant. No fertility specialist could find anything wrong with either of them. All had recommended IVF, which is a common prescription for "unexplained" infertility. By the time they were referred to Toth, they had three failed IVFs under their belts.

He tested both and found the same three bacteria in her cervical culture and his semen. After ten days of IV antibiotics, the bacteria was gone. They wanted to sign up for a fourth IVF. Because the wife was relatively young at thirty-four, Toth advised them to wait six months to give her reproductive system some recovery time. They took a vacation and conceived spontaneously. Today they have two kids, fifteen months apart.

"Even in cases where antibiotic therapy doesn't completely restore fertility, it functions as a *first critical step* in assisting other fertility therapies," claims Toth. In his practice, he found numerous couples who, as it turned out, were both infected with anaerobic bacteria (the kind that don't need oxygen to survive) and mycoplasmas (other bacteria in the reproductive tract), who had undergone multiple ART procedures to no avail. Once treated, they were able to resume fertility drugs and became pregnant after their next try.

Toth discusses another couple who sought him out after two failed IVFs. The wife's tubes were irreparably blocked, so IVF was their last hope. By piecing together their reproductive history, he deduced that the husband had probably infected the wife, who had then developed the PID that had not only ruined her tubes but was preventing her from sustaining a pregnancy resulting from IVF. Toth found two anaerobes and chlamydia in each of their cultures and prescribed ten days of IV antibiotic therapy.

After a three-month wait, instead of the usual six because she was forty-two, they conceived on their next (third) IVF and had a healthy baby boy. This case highlights the most important aspect of any infertility treatment, and that is the need to enlist a couple's cooperation in examining their reproductive histories so the most appropriate therapeutic plan can be created.

Why don't others duplicate his procedures? Toth was too

swamped to give me an interview, but his assistant Connie explained that he feels it's because his approach is preventive and inexpensive and many specialists like to encourage you to take the high-tech, high-priced road. So they don't test for the bacteria, you don't know you have it, and your chances of becoming pregnant are severely compromised. Your chances of conception diminish the longer the bacteria goes undetected.

Lesson #16: If you've got an infection in your reproductive tract, it's almost certain that your partner does too ,and you are not going to get pregnant unless you both clear it up.

And even if you were infection-free when you started trying to conceive, you could have contracted a bacterial infection during infertility surgery, which could negate the entire procedure or affect your ability to carry a child to full term.

It is also possible that during the delivery of a first baby, you could have picked up bacteria that is causing secondary infertility. Where there is blood, there is bacteria.

Believe it or not, antibiotic therapy is still considered experimental. The only way to ensure that Toth's methods become more widespread is by demanding them. Ask your doctor what specific tests have been performed. Don't settle for the standard STD screening, but insist on a deeper probe for other bacteria. If your doctor's lab can't accommodate your request, ask for referrals to a pathologist, one who is willing to incubate the cultures long enough to determine if any other bacteria are present. False-negative responses can occur if the incubation period is too short.

I'd certainly try this route before opening your bank book and submitting to mind-altering drugs and painful procedures with low success rates that could further impair your fertility.

****

Meanwhile, back in Paradise, Jim began fondly referring to the house of my Arizona friends as the "Ashram," and its inhabitants as "the F—king Swammies." When I would come home from trips, revived and renewed, he'd eye me suspiciously. "What'd they do to you? Are you under some kind of spell?"

He thought I was relying too much on them, but couldn't deny that I was well. We headed back to the therapist's office, where I announced that I was never going back to Dr. Casanova.

I couldn't imagine getting back on the infertility roller coaster. Besides, I was at the end of my medical path. I couldn't take any more fertility drugs. Dr. J's operation was now way past the one-year "guarantee." There was a very low success rate for the laparotomy that Dr. Casanova wanted to perform. And with the new house, we didn't have the money at hand for an IVF try. I was not giving up; I was letting go.

Although Jim thought I was "getting too weird," he was relieved that I was off the baby train. In fact, he stated that he wanted to postpone pregnancy for at least another year. I wasn't concerned because I was convinced my baby would come to me when she was ready. But I still wanted to expose Jim to the peace-seeking process, hoping he would derive some benefit. After some gentle coercion, he reluctantly agreed to join me in Arizona for a few days.

Arizona in June is boiling, but the grand house was abundant with light and cheer and awash in gauzy hues. (I went home and painted mine the same colors.) I felt alive with hope, and it felt real.

Jim had decided to quit smoking on the trip, which made him antsy. He also had a hard time slowing down, because as an admitted workaholic (just like his father), he knew no other way. He chose not to be a part of the program except for some hypnosis from Ben for the non-smoking effort. Instead, he raced around in a rented Corvette, listening to Jimi Hendrix. He also told me he was sick of eating "sticks and twigs," his take on vegetarian cuisine. We were definitely out of sync.

He was also afraid my recovery wasn't genuine and worried that I would get sick again. I certainly didn't need him around telling me I was going to drop dead at any minute. By the time he left, I was glad and so was he.

His absence allowed me to immerse myself in my new surroundings, philosophies and friends. I wanted to absorb and incorporate all at once everything they had been studying for years. (I've always prided myself on being a quick study.) Because I was emotionally and spiritually ready, I was able to assimilate a surprising amount of information.

One of the most enduring Life Lessons *Lesson #17 I learned was: GET ON WITH YOUR LIFE AND TRUST THAT THE FUTURE WILL PROVIDE WHAT YOU NEED.*

I learned to change old patterns. I worked on letting go of the *secondary benefits* of illness, like not having to work or always having an out when I didn't want to do something. Lupus had become a convenient excuse. Instead of standing up for myself, I hid behind the disease. I realized that I may have used my illness as a way to get Jim to take care of me. If you ask yourself what you are gaining from your current unhealthy condition, the answers may surprise you.

Each time I rejected an old behavior, I replaced it with a more positive one. (Like exercise instead of alcohol to wind down or making water my beverage of choice all day instead of coffee.)

I changed my thinking and also learned to relax so my thinking *could* change. You should be going for balance here. Your goal is to create your own serenity. You can begin by resting your senses and repositioning and reprogramming your environment.

For example, think about how to make your surroundings as nurturing as possible. You can do this with candlelight, natural light, or twilight and music choices that are soothing. (Almost everyone I know had Pachelbel's Canon played at some point during their wedding. Try that.) Certain colors are more gentle and reassuring, like soft green, or soft pinks. (Don't laugh, but most padded rooms in mental hospitals are in this shade range.) You don't have to paint the house. You can get new sheets. *Lesson #18: Let others help you. Involve well-meaning relatives, who have felt helpless watching you struggle through infertility, in the redecorating and invite them to contribute to the cause.* Also, tranquil visual art can flavor a room as do heartening messages pasted on the bathroom mirror. A particularly promising horoscope goes a long way.

Immerse yourself in a restful, sensual, warm bath (hot ones can be overstimulating) and let it immobilize you in utter relaxation. Think of it as gourmet bathing. Baths are primal. They recreate a womb-like environment.

Walks along the beach, over the hills, and through the woods can be equally settling if you listen for the quiet sounds. And you need the sunlight for the tiny pineal gland, located in the center of the brain, that balances sexual hormones.

If you can't separate yourself from the couch or the bed, bring the sounds of nature into your home. Available now are CD's and tapes composed of rustling trees, crashing waves, wind chimes and rain drops. Close your eyes and get lost. These tapes are also great for maintaining calm, and create an alternative focus for you during ART procedures.

Start screening your phone calls. I never answer the phone anymore. I talk to people only when I want to. My friends are on to me. They holler my name six times and order me to pick up the phone because they think I'm listening. Don't let anyone upset your routine or add to your distress.

The way we breathe air can make a difference. Yogis believe that the mind and breath are enmeshed and that by calming the breath we calm the mind. Ever notice that you have a tendency to hold your breath or breathe shallowly when you are tense?

Years ago I attended a RESOLVE seminar hosted by Dr. Alice Domar and she distributed a handout with "mini-relaxation" exercise instructions, which she gave me permission to reprint here. You will find more detailed variations in her book *Healing Mind, Healthy Woman*.

- Mini-relaxation exercises are focused breathing techniques which help reduce anxiety and tension immediately.
- You can do them with your eyes open or closed.
- You can do them anyplace, at any time. No one will know that you are doing them.

Ways to do a "mini..."

Switch over to diaphragmatic breathing: if you are having trouble, try breathing in through your nose and out through your mouth. You should feel your stomach rising about an inch as you breathe in and falling about an inch as you breathe out. If this is still difficult for you, lie on your back. You will be more aware of your breathing pattern. Remember it is impossible to breathe diaphragmatically if you are holding in your stomach! So relax your stomach muscles.

Mini Version 1

Count (backward) very slowly to yourself from ten to zero, one number for each breath. Thus, with the first diaphragmatic breath, you say "ten" to yourself. With the next breath, you say "nine," etc. If you start feeling light-headed or dizzy, slow down the counting. When you get to "zero," see how you are feeling. If you're not feeling better, try doing it again.

Mini Version 2

As you inhale, count very slowly up to four; as you exhale, count slowly back to one. Thus, as you inhale, you say to yourself, "one, two, three, four." As you exhale, you say to yourself, "four, three, two, one." Do this several times.

Mini Version 3

After each inhalation, pause for a few seconds. After you exhale, pause again for a few seconds. Do this for several breaths.

Good times to "do a mini"

When you're stuck in traffic...when you're put on hold during important call...when you're waiting in your doctor's office...when someone says something that bothers you...whenever you're at a red light...when you're waiting for a phone call...when you're in the dentist's chair...when you're feeling overwhelmed by what you need to accomplish in the near future...when you're standing in line...when you're in pain...etc,... THE ONLY TIME THAT MINIS DO NOT WORK IS WHEN YOU FORGET TO DO THEM!

I also practiced alternate nostril breathing, which gave me a natural high. Cover the right nostril and deeply inhale through the left one. Then cover the left one and fully exhale through the right. Deeply inhale through the right, while covering the left. Cover the right and exhale through the left. Repeat ten times daily. When you're feeling especially bottled up, you can practice the "breath of fire," as it is known in kundalini yoga. Take a deep breath and blow as forcefully as you can in rapid bursts. Repeat six times. You will feel cleared immediately.

There are many kinds of yoga, but kundalini, meaning the energy of creation, is noted for the speed with which it works, according to Sat Jivan Kaur Khalsa, a New York city kundalini yoga instructor who devotes a good portion of her practice to successfully treating infertility clients. The symbol for kundalini is the serpent; and by moving energy, you uncoil the snake. "By combining techniques from all the different branches of yoga, kundalini takes the energy that everyone has and moves it for healing and awareness," says Khalsa. "It wakes you up!"

She claims that this type of yoga works *very quickly* on the glandular (endocrine) system, beginning with the pituitary gland. By using specific sound, movement, and the breath, she can "lessen the stress that tampers with the reproductive system." Anna DeLury, a Los Angeles yoga instructor with a B.S. in Kinesiology, told me the same thing. "Stress is a legitimate factor that can cause infertility."

In addition to relaxing ovaries, Khalsa said she can dramatically increase male potency by prescribing strenuous exercises, including many frog poses. She also told me that fresh garlic increases sexual energy in both sexes, and advocates adding it to everything.

Khalsa pointed out that while it is important to prepare on a physical level to conceive, you must not forget that you are trying to bring into the world a soul as well. "Although pregnancy manifests physically, the couple must also attract the baby's soul energy," she explained. Khalsa can be reached directly at (212) 995-0571 or call the International Kundalini Yoga Teachers' Association for a referral at (505) 753-0423.

It's difficult to achieve the full benefit of yoga from a book or tape, but if you want to get started, try *Kundalini Yoga: The Flow of Eternal Power* by Shakti Parwha Kaur Khalsa (Time Capsule Books, 1996). It has great illustrations and recipes. Also, yoga audio tapes are available from The Mind/Body Medical Institute at (617) 632-9525.

Since my friend Renee knew that it took sperm at least five to twenty minutes to reach the uterus and fallopian tubes, she stood on her head for half an hour after intercourse while her husband held up her legs. She turned on the television to distract him from the flattering angle at which she was posed. Gary Collins and Sarah Purcell were on the now defunct "Home Show" interviewing women who had children but would not want them if they had to do it all over again. How inspiring.

Tony Robbins, the motivational speaker and success peddler, says when asked how he got so successful, "The same thing that drives all of us to succeed: Inspiration or desperation."

It was pure desperation that made me finally break down and exercise. I started in Arizona. (It was the first real workout I'd had since high-school cheerleading, unless you count running my mouth or taking Alex to the vet.) I was literally twitching from all my stress.

You don't have to join a gym for this. The goal is inner calmness, not rippling muscles. Renee swears by her treadmill. I jumped madly on my mini-trampoline. I could only manage seven-minute sessions at first, but within a month I was up to thirty minutes a day, five days a week. And I didn't need a $90 outfit to work out. *Lesson #19: What you do need is underwear that fits. You don't need to be constantly measuring yourself against those teeny briefs you ordered from the Victoria's Secret catalogue that only fit store mannequins. Go buy some that are comfortable, snip out the size, and start exercising!*

You don't really need equipment, either. Take to the streets. When I walked with Alex around the neighborhood to commune with nature, I went incognito, intent on getting a good workout without neighborly interruptions. He always gave me away, though, because there were no other Weimaraners in the vicinity and he was exceptionally noisy. Another dog's appearance was grounds for maniacal barking and body thrashing. (But he was terrified of our vacuum cleaner.) I got some thoracic benefit by wrestling him back on to the sidewalk where we resumed our brisk clip until another creature violated his space.

Regarding the health benefits that come from caring for animals, studies show that when people are interacting with their animals their blood pressure decreases significantly. Cats (not kittens) are also relaxing pals. I had a lovable ten-year-old Siamese named Sasha, who was my bed buddy. (He went to heaven in July 1997 at the age of eighteen. I dearly miss him.) Animals love you no matter what. You can express your emotions and receive unconditional love. Besides, they don't have much memory capacity, except for where their food is kept and their feeding time, and they like the taste of tears.

While exercising with or without your four-legged friends, remember that exercise can also increase sexual desire. In a 1994 *Glamour* article entitled "How Exercise Can Make Your Sex Life Soar," stress was credited as one of the most common causes of sexual dysfunction. Sex therapist Jo Marie Kessler says "Exercise helps reduce the internal chatter that can distract you. It's hard to get your genitals to respond when your brain (is elsewhere)."

In the same article, James White, Ph.D., professor emeritus of P.E. at UCSD explains, "Sex is a physical activity. Exercise puts you in better physical shape to be sexual." According to psychologist and sex therapist Linda De Villers, Ph.D., of Santa Monica, CA, "Exercise also raises body temperatures, causing the brain's hypothalamus to produce alpha waves." These waves relax muscles and release tension, leaving you more receptive to sexual thoughts and actions. She concludes, "Exercise gives women a second sexual wind." (I needed a gale force.)

But it's well documented that too much exercise as well as too much body fat can impair fertility. Women who are thin or excessively athletic often experience decreased estrogen levels, which interferes with ovulation and menstruation cycles. Obese women produce too much estrogen, which also causes menstrual irregularities. (The clinical definition of "obese" is only thirty pounds overweight!) *Lesson #20: Close your eyes when they routinely weigh you at each doctor's appointment. Why let those inaccurately high scales ruin your day? This is called healthy denial.* Thinness in men can result in low sperm counts, and male obesity impedes healthy sperm production. Weight levels in both partners "should be addressed before (introducing) hormone treatment," according to G. William Bates, M.D., vice president of medical education and research of Greenville Hospital Systems in South Carolina as reported in *Prevention* magazine's "Healing with Vitamins" (Rodale Press, 1996.)

I figured that what you put in your mouth could affect your fertility, but I could find no existing, specific nutritional recipe for combatting infertility. Nutritional prescriptions abound for every kind of malady imaginable except this one. My friend and colleague, Stephen Sinatra, M.D., F.A.C.C., helped me to formulate an infertility regimen for the purposes of this book, and I rounded out his research with some of my other findings.

Board certified in internal medicine, cardiology, and bioenergetic psychotherapy, Dr. Sinatra is the author of *Optimum Health: A Natural Lifesaving Prescription for Your Body and Mind* (Bantam Books, 1996). The following recommended doses are for *both* men and women. This is because a deficiency in any one of these areas can upset the body's delicate balance and sabotage your ability to conceive either naturally or with low- or high-tech assistance.

AMINO ACIDS are the building blocks of protein, which you need for hormone development and libido. Good sources for protein are eggs, fish, poultry, and soy products. Some amino acids, as growth hormone precursors, need to be added to ensure the adequate production of sex hormones. *L-arginine with L-ornithine* should be taken before exercise and before bed. Dose: 750 mg three times daily. *L-glutamine* dose: 500 mg three times daily.

ESSENTIAL FATTY ACIDS are also necessary for peak hormonal performance. EFA rich foods with *Alpha-linolenic acid* are tofu, grapeseed oil, wheat germ, oatmeal, and nuts like walnuts. Fish also provides good sources of EPA and DHA, which are Omega-3 Essential Fatty Acids.

Vitamins

Coenzyme Q10 enables men with hypospermia (low sperm count) to impregnate women by increasing sperm motility.

Coenzyme Q10 can rescue any tissue in need. Although there is no data to support its use in women yet, because of its effectiveness in men it is also recommended for women. Dose: 30 mg three times daily after meals.

Vitamin E surfaced in many references as a fertility promoter. It stimulates prostaglandins, which are needed to turn on the reproductive hormones, and helps prevent miscarriages and premature births. Dose: 400-800 IUs daily.

Folic Acid has been shown to reduce the frequency of birth defects and cervical cancer. Dose: 800 mcg daily.

Vitamin C keeps sperm moving. Low levels of Vitamin C cause sperm to clump together. (This is easily diagnosed because it can be seen under a microscope.) Dose: 500 mg twice daily. Because studies have shown that smoking cigarettes depletes the body of vitamin C, extra C is important for smokers.

Multi B-complex supplements are necessary, especially if alcohol and caffeine are used. Dose: 20-40 mg per day.

Zinc helps testosterone production and helps prevent prostate problems. Pumpkin seeds, seafood, beef, lamb, wheat germ, miso and whole grains are good dietary sources. Men need extra for sexual vigor. Dose: 30 mg daily.

Foods

Sesame Seeds are richer in calcium than dairy products, richer in protein than meat, and can be eaten in the form of sesame butter, humus, or tahini.

Honey is packed with amino acids, several vitamins and minerals, and is great energy food and natural sweetener.

Kelp is loaded with iodine, which is needed for a healthy thyroid, a gland crucial in the production of sexual hormones. Kelp can be sprinkled on soups and salads.

Eggs and Soybeans are a good source for lecithin, which is found in the endocrine glands most important for reproduction. It is also necessary for the production of semen.

Seaweed repairs tissues, builds new cells, and helps with sex hormone production. One teaspoon daily.

Garlic balances the endocrine glands and helps restore the balance for glandular disorders. Fresh is best, a bulb at a meal, or it can be taken in *Kyolic* tablets, which are high quality and deodorized.

Cranberry, Blackberry, and Cherry juices can facilitate reproductive function.

Dr. Stephen Sinatra's Phytoestrogen Infertility Shake:

Grind two tbsp. of flaxseed in your coffee grinder and mix with an 8 oz. glass of vanilla flavored soy milk. Drink daily.

Daily Herbs

Red Clover Flowers, a member of the pea/bean family, have a high content of protein, calcium, and magnesium which benefit the entire body. They balance the acid/alkaline level of the vagina and uterus to favor conception. Fresh flowers can be added to salad. Dried flowers can be cooked with rice. Can also be taken as a tea.

Red Raspberry Leaves promote uterine function and sperm motility. They are most effective when combined with Red Clover. Contains calcium and magnesium, whose levels are depleted by alcohol, sugar, and caffeine. Can be taken as tea.

Stinging Nettles help uterine, kidney, and hormonal function. Dose: 1/4 tsp. of fresh or dried seeds. Can be taken as tea, one or more cups per day. Can be continued to help sustain pregnancy.

Dong Quai Root normalizes menstrual periods. It should only be taken the second two weeks of the cycle during ovulation and menstruation. Sold as a water-based extract under the name of "Tang Kwei Gin." Best used in conjunction with above herbs. Add 5-25 drops to above mentioned teas.

False Unicorn Root is a uterine tonic for those prone to miscarriage. It has an alkaline effect on ovaries, kidneys, and bladder and is taken as a tincture or extract. Add 5-15 drops to water or tea.

Saw Palmetto promotes healthy prostate function. Dose: 200 mg daily.

Alfalfa, parsley, watercress, and dandelion leaves have properties that promote sexual function. Add to salads or use while cooking.

According to author Susun S. Weed, in her book *Herbal for the Childbearing Year* (Ash Tree Publishing, 1986), "*Lunaception* combines well with herbs that promote fertility." She reasons that since ovulation is controlled by light, you should leave a light on in your bedroom for three days midway through your menstrual cycle. All other nights, you should keep your bedroom in total darkness. She says you will ovulate when the light is on and should make love during the three "light" nights in order to conceive.

Pulsatilla is one of a number of homeopathic remedies that may be used, under the care of a licensed homeopathic practitioner, to treat infertility. Call Homeopathic Educational Services, in Berkeley, California, (510) 649-0294 to order a national directory of homeopathic nurses and MDs.

The following sources were also used in compiling the nutritional guidelines of this book:

Christine Anderson, D.C., D.I.C.C.P., Los Angeles

Food and Healing by Annemarie Colbin, Ballantine Books (1996)

Prevention's Healing with Vitamins by Earl Dawson, M.D., Ph.D., associate professor of OB/GYN, University of Texas Medical School at Galveston, Rodale Press (1996)

Love, Sex and Nutrition by Bernard Jensen, D.C., (1988)

Healing Wise by Susun S. Weed. Ash Tree Publishing, (1989)

It's worth noting that water should be taken liberally to flush the system and to keep bodily functions in gear. Make sure it is not distilled, or it will carry too many minerals away from the body.

from feeling sluggish and blocked. There is widespread belief today among holistic healers that trapped energy acts as a conception barrier and short-circuits the natural energy flow.

"To achieve sexual health, any blockages or toxic accumulations which impede the flow of energy must be dissolved..." say Michio and Aveline Kushi, authors of *Macrobiotic Pregnancy and Care of the Newborn* (Japan Publications, 1984). They believe most people suffer from various degrees of stagnation around the intestinal region and reproductive organs, which can dull desire and sexual activity.

Once you streamline your diet, another way to get unblocked is with chiropractic realignment. Dr. Christine Anderson, a Los Angeles-based chiropractor who is board-certified in pediatrics and pregnancy, states that mental stress causes spinal misalignment and spinal misalignment causes infertility. You may not know you are out of alignment. "People think because they're not in pain, they don't have a problem," says Dr. Anderson, "You can have the problem before you have the pain."

You can experience different types of infertility depending on where your vertebral misalignment or subluxation is located. Cranial subluxation of the first cervical vertebra, for example, can affect the blood flow to the pituitary gland and therefore interfere with healthy hormonal activity. The twelfth thoracic vertebra in the lower mid-back controls ovarian, tubal, and uterine function in women and testicular and penile function in men. Adjusting the part of the spine that controls and coordinates reproductive function increases the essential nerve and blood supply to the reproductive organs.

If you are out of alignment, high-tech procedures may have little chance of being successful. Chiropractic measures should be sought out early, before you are broke and broken down.

"My treatments have made pregnancy possible!" claims Dr. Anderson.

And the process isn't long or expensive. Three visits per

week for two months, at a cost of $50 per visit, are covered by most insurance plans. For referrals of doctors specifically trained in infertility and pregnancy, call The International Chiropractors' Association Council on Chiropractic Pediatrics at (703) 528-5000. Dr. Anderson can be reached at (213) 467-6348.

In his book *Healing and the Mind* (Doubleday, 1993), Bill Moyers talked with Dr. David Eisenberg, the first American medical student sent to China in 1979, now an instructor at the Harvard Medical School, who elaborated on acupuncture's solution for untrapping energy. "The body is made up of channels or circuits that apply to each organ through which the energy flows, and this energy has to be in balance...The acupuncture treatment clears energy imbalances...and when the passages are clear, the energy will flow and the patient will recover."

Dr. Daoshing Ni, L.Ac., D.O.M., Ph.D., of the Union of Tao and Man Traditional Acupuncture, Inc. in Santa Monica, CA, told me that half of his practice is devoted to reproductive medicine. He sees about 2500 infertility patients per year, mostly women, whom he treats with Traditional Chinese Medicine (TCM): acupuncture, accupressure, massage, manipulation, and herbs. For each individual, he creates a treatment plan to change their neurological responses and solicit their endorphins and natural healing chemicals. His program also jump-starts the body's sluggish reaction to fertility drugs, regulates hormone levels, and reduces the thinning of the uterine lining that often results from chlomid. For men, TCM can improve semen analysis, and for both, TCM can increase vitality and libido.

"Stress causes infertility," Dr. Daoshing Ni states emphatically. Donna Georgakopoulos, L. Ac., Dipl. Ac., of Burbank, CA, agrees. "Many physical barriers to infertility can have emotional foundations. Everything is interconnected." TCM works wonders with crazed patients who need calming and de-stress-

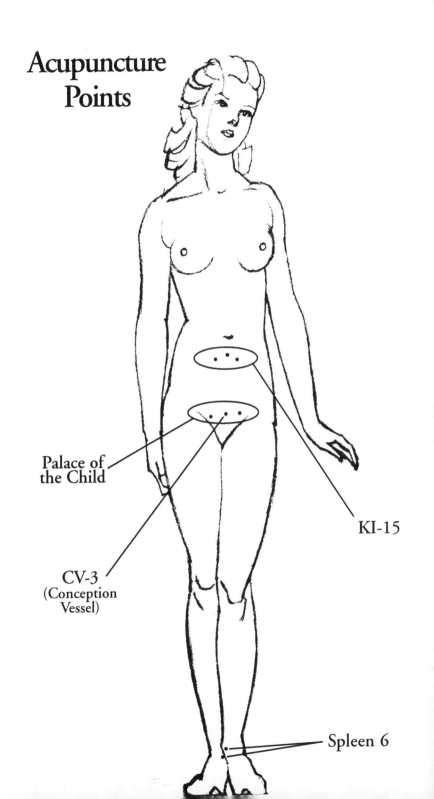

Acupuncture
Points

Palace of
the Child

KI-15

CV-3
(Conception
Vessel)

Spleen 6

ing. But the older you are and the longer you have suffered infertility, the more resistant to reversal your condition can be. Dr. Daoshing Ni laments that most patients seek him out as a last resort after years of unsuccessful conventional infertility treatments and ART.

He advocates an *integrative* approach combining Chinese and Western medicines to enhance the odds and increase the likelihood of successful conception.

The TCM method consists of weekly visits for three to eighteen months, at a cost of approximately $100 per week. For a licensed doctor in your area, contact the American Association of Acupuncture and Oriental Medicine at (610) 266-1433, 433 Front Street, Catasauqua, PA 18032.

You or your husband can do accupressure on yourself. Scottsdale, AZ chiropractor, Dr. Roberta Vaseleniuck, showed me how you could "turn on" your "Palace of the Child." Rub CV-3, the conception vessel, and the pressure points on either side of it. They are centered just above the public bone (see diagram), and should be massaged daily with four fingers laterally. Daily stroking in a straight line from below the pubic bone all the way up to your lower lip, is another way to activate the conception vessel.

If you have uterine or tubal problems, apply medium pressure to the KI-15 area of the abdomen. And for "female" problems of any kind, the Spleen six points above the inner ankles should be massaged (*See chart on theprevious page.*)

The world is rampant with old wives' tales about how to conceive, like having a baby pee on your bed. And some new ones, like drinking cough medicine to change cervical mucus. (Renee had her pregnant sister, Rose, "Spread her aura" around her house.) I found a charming book called *Mothers of Thyme* by Janet L. Sha (Lida Rose Press, 1990), chock full of old customs and fertility rituals.

One of the most amusing pieces of folkloric disinformation

blamed infertility on too much "brainwork." In the late 1800's, women were being educated in record numbers. It was thought that because the women were expanding their brains with knowledge, they were depriving the "menstrual organs" of their "nervepower." A study conducted during this period confirmed the worst: "Of the 705 women who went to college, only 196 married and of those, only sixty-six had children."

Some of the prescribed "cures" seemed almost a punishment for being infertile. Native American women from northeast California were forced to wear little gray birds, alive, under their clothing and Aowin women from South Ghana were subjected to a powdered white clay douche followed by a pepper or ginger enema.

I'll pause here in case you need to sneeze...You will need your nasal passages fully cleared to appreciate the primitive and potent part the sense of smell plays in your overall well-being.

The *Los Angeles Times* featured an article by Sheryl Stolberg in June 1994, about the science of smell, and about Dr. Alan Hirsch, who is a Chicago neurologist treating people with olfactory disorders. "But his passion," states Stolberg, "is investigating the murky arena of how smells affect behavior." More specifically, he wanted to know what scents turned men on. (My first guess would be new car smell.)

The only scent that consistently gorged men's genitals (measured by monitors to detect increased blood flow) was fresh-baked cinnamon buns. But before you start rubbing cinnamon behind your ears, you may want to stop by the bakery instead. Consider Hirsch's conclusion: "The way to a man's heart really is through his stomach."

Hirsch also says, "Smell has the most powerful impact of any sense." He has conducted experiments to prove his point. One involved gamblers who plunked forty-five percent more quarters into slot machines when a Las Vegas casino was scented with a pleasant artificial smell. When Hirsch increased the odor level, he found spending increased fifty-three percent. (Spray your husband with eau de cologne while he's balancing the checkbook.)

Even the old medical guard has signed on. At Memorial Sloan-Kettering Cancer Center in New York, doctors are using a relaxing vanilla scent to calm patients undergoing stressful MRIs.

In her article, Stolberg relates that there is good scientific reason to believe that smell has the power to shape emotions and behavior. Neurologist Richard Costanza, an olfactory researcher at the Medical College of Virginia explains that vision, hearing, and touch travel a convoluted path to the limbic system, the emotional center of the brain. But smell and taste are directly wired to it. When a scent is inhaled, it travels through the nostrils to the olfactory bulb, which fires a fast message to the limbic system. "Smell and taste... have a more privileged access (to the brain.)" Costanzo says.

In her book *Complete Aromatherapy Handbook: Essential Oils for Radiant Health* (Sterling Publishing, 1990), Susanne Fischer-Rizzi discusses how pleasing fragrances stimulate the limbic system, the seat of our sexuality, motivation, and moods, to release neurotransmitters helpful to conception—among them encephaline, endorphins and serotonin. Encephaline and endorphins, reduce pain and produce a feeling of well-being. Endorphins also stimulate sexual feelings, while serotonin helps relax and calm.

Certain aromas elicit certain responses and are used for specific reasons. Read on for Fischer-Rizzi's fertility aids.

Jasmine (plant or oil—not to be taken orally) is used as a cramp reliever and uterine tonic, and as an antidepressant and aphrodisiac. Jasmine has been traditionally used for impotence, frigidity, back pain, depression, fear, pessimism, and emotional suffering. "No other essential oil is quite as capable of changing our mood so intensely. Jasmine oil offers little choice other than optimism...(and) is especially helpful for emotional dilem-mas...(involving) relationships and sex." Dilute the oil, because the gentler the fragrance, the more effective it will be. (So much for drowning yourself in it. The "more is better" theory doesn't apply here.)

Chamomile is for the cranky, discontented, and impatient among us. It is calming and tension relieving and helps reduce anger, insomnia, oversensitivity, and depression. Chamomile is a stomach soother and counteracts morning sickness. The rec-ommended oral dosage is two to three drops, diluted, three times daily. Or you can add it to your bath or put it on a lamp with a cotton ball.

Patchouli oil, toxic when ingested, acts as an aphrodisiac and may also be added to the bath, or body lotion, or to a light bulb.

Oil of Rose balances things out of kilter, particularly prob-lems related to the heart. "Rose oil comforts in times of sorrow, dissolves psychological pain, refreshes a sad heart and opens doors to love, friendship, and empathy." It also may gently dissolve blockages and feelings of disappointment or depres-sion. The result is gentle balance. Make sure you get authentic rose oil, not an imitation. Demand oil made from rose plants—Rosa damascena, Rosa centifolia, or Rose gallica. Put one or two drops on a light bulb or add to your bath.

(Ahhhh...feeling languid or lazy yet?)

Recalling a particularly stellar moment in your life can also uplift you when you're in the dumps. This always works for me.

Think of a time when you felt especially loved or lov-ing... Relive it for minutes on end.

Think of a time when you triumphed over adver-sity...Relive it for minutes on end.

Think of a time of simple joy felt in childhood, adoles-cence or adulthood...Relive these moments.

One time I felt especially loved was in tenth grade when my

mother surprised me with a pair of new slippers because I'd gotten my first part—(the second lead)—in the school play. They were fluffy and pink, and I awoke to find them at the foot of my bed.

A moment of great triumph for me was making the junior varsity cheerleading squad as a freshman. From over a hundred girls that tried out, only two of us were selected. As I relived these and other moments, I could still feel the joy and satisfaction they had brought. They gave me hope that there were more happy moments to come.

And of course when all else fails, you can go shopping. I have a friend who blurted out one of the darker female secrets by admitting to her husband at the height of a fight, "I just need to go to the mall for an hour and I'll be all right."

Lesson #21: Treating yourself, not to a shopping binge, which can cause a financial hangover, but to a one-time diversion like a special sweater, etc., can give you an energy lift. So can a new book. Whether it's a form of escape, or an inspirational self-help, it's an inexpensive way to take care of yourself.

If you're still feeling blocked, a trip through the mall can also get the sexual juices flowing. My therapist told me that women with certain fetishes can have an orgasm just by touching luxury items. Time to go to Bloomingdale's and start stroking those Anne Klein pumps. What a boost. Whew.

Sex life need a little spark? (How about a bonfire?) Feeling a little dulled? *Lesson #22: Start with yourself.* Masturbation, otherwise delicately known as "self-exploration," is one way to get back into the swing of things. Studies show that women who masturbate even once a month have more sexual desire, take less time to be aroused, and have greater sexual satisfaction with their partners. (I must confess that I didn't get the hang of it until I was twenty-six and used the boomer bible, *Our Bodies, Ourselves* as a roadmap. I was stifled early—age six—when my mother walked into my room and found me "exploring." She hastily informed me that my body was a temple of the Holy Spirit and that particular area belonged to Him and I'd better leave it alone. I did. For twenty years. Now I thank Him when I'm done. *Lesson #23: It's not where you start, it's where you finish.*

If you are uncomfortable with or feel ill-informed about masturbation, there is only one book you'll ever need. *Sex for One: The Joy of Selfloving* by Betty Dodson, Ph.D., (Three Rivers Press, 1996) normalizes the subject with information and acceptance. The book features plainspoken prose and explicit diagrams for beginners as well as old hands. Masturbation isn't only to be practiced alone. Dodson presents masturbation as a prelude to "partnersex" as well.

To stir up your own sexual juices, I found a trilogy of books (in paperback at most bookstores) called *The Erotic Adventures of Sleeping Beauty* by Anne Rice writing as A.N. Roquelaure, (Penguin Books, 1985). The book jacket states that each is "An erotic novel of discipline, love, and surrender...A teasing exploration of the psychology of human desire." I can tell you that it's HOT stuff.

When sex became a chore for one couple I know, the husband would start masturbating without his wife. Then he would call her in at the last minute and she would jump on just in time.

Helping your guy along can become part of your ritual. The Los Angeles-based sex educator and creator of "The Sexuality Seminars," which she presents internationally, L. Lou Paget offers some pointers. She told me that for the majority of men, the most sensitive part of the penis is the quarter-sized area on the underside at the base of the tip. It's shaped like a V and it's called the frenulum. She also gave the following suggestions for incorporating oral and manual stimulation as a way to build his excitement more easily.

• Your tongue is *always* in motion.

- Your teeth are covered or artfully applied.
- Your hand is an extension of your mouth. They work in concert with each other.
- Your free hand is building sensation elsewhere.
- Your mouth is not a vacuum.

Instead of your mouth, you can use both hands with a good lubricant. If lubricants are permissible, Paget likes Astroglide, which is clear, water-based, tasteless, and available at most drugstores.

Also, Femme Productions brings you the first video pornography by women, for women, about women and men, rentable in most video stores. And there's a new sex cable channel for women called "Adam & Eve," which features soft porn and no violence or S & M.

If you don't want to brave the sex shoppes, (I confess I didn't, although the women in my therapy group said it's very empowering), try phone or mail order. (I preferred hiding in my bedroom and dialing after a glass of wine.)

I found a great store in San Francisco called Good Vibrations at (800) 289-8423, that offers sex toys and "previously banned" books by catalogue. (I discovered them in *Glamour* magazine, which I consider pretty homogenized.) You can give them the product numbers so you don't have to mention the items by name. I saw a lot of mysterious devices that had potential. The catalogue explains where to put what, in light, playful descriptions. They also mail everything in plain wrapper and vow never to sell a list with your name on it.

If you're not feeling perked up yet, you may need to do some anger-release work. According to my therapist, "Depression is the energy reduction that comes from suppressing your feelings. It is anger turned inward." A psychic friend of mine once claimed, "Anger can burn down buildings or launch rocket ships." So blow out the negative stuff and use the energy to throw yourself into something positive.

One recipe for getting rid of pent-up anger is driving around in the car (windows up) and screaming for all you're worth. Another remedy is screaming with a pillow over your face. Punching bed pillows is also rather satisfying. But my favorite tool is the plastic baseball bat that I originally purchased as a training tool for Alex. The trainer said to bop him on the top of his head to give him a correction. It never really worked, and I felt so bad when I did it that I'd cuddle him immediately afterward. I think he found the mixed messages confusing. (Besides, once he was neutered, he was a little less rambunctious. Jim had beseeched me not to "cut his balls off," but I stood firm. "Can't he get laid just once?" Jim begged, obviously sharing some gender identification with Alex. I gave him the lecture about bringing unwanted puppies into the world and tried to appeal to his social conscience, but he kept grabbing his crotch and making faces at me. I remained unfazed, but assured him I would wait until he was away on business.) Anyway, the bat really wears you out. And if you incorporate yelling into your routine, it's a great way to purge yourself of anxiety. Just keep pounding on the bed until you're hoarse.

Pounding a punching bag is one sure way to beat the blues. At Billy Blank's World Training Center in Sherman Oaks, CA, women's boxing is catching on. You can release a lifetime of aggression by throwing punches with a trainer, who's praising you and won't hit you back. You'll learn mental and physical awareness and you can keep boxing throughout your entire pregnancy.

More suggestions from formerly angry women: Scrub the kitchen floor. (This wasn't one of my methods. I'd rather have a root canal than clean the house.) Yell into paper bags and pop them. If you're a thrower, try firing ice cubes into the shower or tub. If you need to demolish things, make sure it's stuff you have handy but don't care about, like newspapers to shred or pencils to snap. Sophia likes to break plates (she's Greek) but since most of us don't have several sets of dinnerware, use the old Corelle ware. (That's the only thing in my kitchen that survived the earthquake.) Kneading dough can be satisfying, and you'll have something to enjoy and feed your friends when you're done.

One of my therapist's favorite damage control tips is to write the name of the person you are most upset with on the bottom of your running shoes. You'll get satisfaction with each smack of the pavement.

Another remedy for letting old anger go is to write a letter to the person who wronged you, and set it on fire. I had a really bad boss once, and writing was the only way to get rid of the fury I felt because of the injustices suffered at his hands. When you write, you get the mess out of your head and onto paper; then you have a tangible representation of your rage and you can do something physical to make it go away.

You don't have to set all your writing on fire. You can start journaling. The journal acts as a receptacle for your frustrations and feelings, and the act of unburdening yourself often gives way to new clarity. I've used this tool for years.

Sometimes you just need to wail. Do not do this with your partner. Call a good friend and preface your remarks with exactly what you want from them: 'I just want to vent,' or 'I just need to dump.' Instruct them not to problem-solve, just to listen and make appropriate, supportive, monosyllabic sounds intermittently so you know they are still on the line.

One way to get some time out for yourself and your partner is to laugh. Norman Cousins used laughter to ease the pain from his rare collagen disease and discovered he not only felt better, he actually improved his health. He asked family and friends to supply him with funny material like the Marx brothers' movies, and he quite literally laughed himself well. At the time, he was the only known survivor of his illness. You can entertain yourselves and foster your own healing with the old "Saturday Night Live" reruns, for instance, or try some of my favorite comedies and feel-good films listed below. This is easy homework with instantaneous results.

Comedies:	*Feel-Good Movies*:
Adams Rib	An Officer and a Gentleman
All About Bob	Annie Hall
Beetlejuice	The Big Chill
Being There	Chariots of Fire
Beverly Hills Cop I	Cool Runnings
Caddyshack	Dominick and Eugene
A Fish Called Wanda	Flashdance
Hannah and Her Sisters	Forrest Gump
Midnight Run	Fried Green Tomatoes
Moonstruck	The Goodbye Girl
My Cousin Vinny	Homeward Bound
Naked Gun	Ice Castles
The Princess Bride	Places in the Heart
Prizzi's Honor	Pretty Woman
Sister Act	Ramblin' Rose
Soapdish	Rudy
Trading Places	Shirley Valentine
Tootsie	Stand and Deliver
Young Frankenstein	This is My Life
	Working Girl

A good cry cleanses the soul. If you are having trouble releasing the tears, watch a tender movie that will turn on the faucets. For pure escape, try the Spellbinders.

And, of course, anything with Barbra Streisand. (Except for that dumb boxing movie with Ryan O'Neal.)

Spellbinders:	*Tear-jerkers*:
Body Heat	An Affair to Remember
Charade	Backstreet
Dead Again	Brian's Song
Dial M for Murder	Casablanca
The Fugitive	Ghost
No Way Out	My Left Foot
Presumed Innocent	Time Flies When You're Alive
Rear Window	The Way We Were
Spellbound	West Side Story
To Catch a Thief	Who's Life is it Anyway?

Other ways to un-slump yourself: Laurel said that gardening made her feel more fertile because she was making things grow. Sophia's sister took up ice skating. Besides the physical exhilaration, she met a bunch of women who weren't privy to her infertility history, and had a ball.

Been bowling lately? It's back in fashion. You can get a real bang out of smashing pins and high scores. If I sound smug, it's because I've actually broken 100—once. (I also broke three nails, which really ticked me off, so I only bowl now when I need a manicure.)

Then for the radical few: You can alter your appearance. This is an old staple of mine. I love the beauty parlor. Experimenting with hair color and cuts can be a great diversion. I've been everything from dark chestnut to shimmery blonde, curly perms to stick straight, elbow length to cropped short. My hairdresser, Germaine, genuflects whenever I walk into the salon. I could have a Master's degree for what I've spent, but then I'd just have a piece of paper instead of those fond memories of shocking friends and confusing acquaintances, who can't quite place me from one coif to the next. (Once the kid comes, you'll have no time for such fancies, so best enjoy them while you can.)

If you can find the will to make some changes, you will be richly rewarded emotionally and physically. I still wasn't pregnant, and that was my ultimate goal, but while I was waiting, I was living again. My body felt healthier. I was in a better place to make decisions. And I found some peace. Deep in my heart, I knew I was steps closer to my baby.

CHAPTER V

MIND BENDING

"When we talk to God, we're praying. When God talks to us, we're schizophrenic."
                                                        —Lily Tomlin

One of Jim's favorite excursions in Arizona was a trip to a crystal shop. I had read that rose quartz crystals promoted fertility, and I was searching for just the right one. Jim was hissing at my heels about the cost, but luckily they were among the more affordable stones. Sophia was weaving around with several finds, totaling in the hundreds. Ben picked up a rose quartz, held it firmly and said "This rock is very powerful. It will make someone pregnant." I ripped it out of his hands and put my $20 on the counter. Sold! Since the rock was pink, I was more convinced that our future child would be a girl. I told Jim I wanted to name her Rose. "I'm not naming a kid after a rock!" He was adamant.

Renee pinned a small crystal (from me) to her underwear during the day and to her comforter at night. She also kept a larger one (also from me) by the bed. *Lesson #24: Crystals are not transferable. If you get pregnant, that crystal belongs to the child. Buy your girlfriend her own. They make great gifts.* It took Renee nearly two years to investigate alternatives outside the doctor's office. She just couldn't shake her belief in the medical profession. After repeated failures, however, her desperation overtook her skepticism, and she opened herself to nontraditional options.

I was way ahead of Renee, convinced I had a direct pipeline to the world beyond. I was talking to everyone at this point and they were talking back to me. I prayed to and received responses from Robert, who I considered my intercessor with God, my old friend the Holy Spirit, and my new spirit guide, Edward. (More on how I found him later.) A January 1995 poll in *Newsweek* showed ninety percent of people believe in God, so I feel I'm on safe ground here. Prayer is a good, simple way to go. I don't necessarily mean Hail Marys or Our Fathers, just talking to God. The shower is my favorite praying place. I always imagine that the water is the white light of God and He is showering me with His grace. If it's okay to talk to animals and plants, not to mention yourself, (I do most of this self-dialogue in the grocery store, where I have lots of company), then why not talk to those who reside in the next plane?

What do we really know, so far, about how prayer may positively affect the course of illness? The question of how spirituality relates to health is taboo to many medical doctors. Nevertheless, there are over one hundred controlled, scientifically sound experiments in the medical literature examining prayer's role in healing.

One of the best guides through the hotly debated area of prayer's role in medicine is Larry Dossey, M.D., the current co-chairman of the Panel on Mind/Body Interventions, Office of Alternative Medicine, National Institute of Health. In his book *Healing Words: The Power of Prayer and The Practice of Medicine* (Harper San Francisco, 1993), Dossey's survey of the medical literature on prayer turns up the surprising fact that *there appears to be no right way to pray*. He does, however, recount the findings of the Spindrift Organization in Oregon, which has spent over a decade conducting low-tech laboratory experiments proving that prayer works. Spindrift has also explored which type of prayer approach seems to yield the most effective outcome. Their researchers studied both "directed" and "non-directed" prayer and came up with some compelling results.

Directed prayer consists of praying with a specific goal or outcome in mind. It is an active attempt to produce specific results. For example, those in directed prayer may be praying for a cessation of a shingles attack, the remission of a cancer or the resolution of a chronic sinus infection. Non-directed prayer, however, involves an open-minded petition with no precise goal. In a sense, the practitioner places ultimate trust in their God or Fate by asking for the best possible outcome to prevail in their life.

Dossey notes that while Spindrift found both directed and non-directed methods effective, the non-directed prayers frequently produced results that were at least twice as successful as the results of direct prayers. These findings aside, Dossey points out that there are simply too many variables and mysteries involved in illness and healing to prescribe what kinds of prayers seem most likely to cure a given medical condition. To my knowledge, there are no clinical studies examining the effects of prayer on infertility. But it seems just a matter of time before savvy mind/body researchers make the application. As infertility is a complex and mysterious condition, you have everything to gain by practicing conscious prayer of any kind. Remember, prayer is a proven route to better mind/body health, and it can definitely help you through your journey.

I think my praying and chanting was getting to Jim. I would jump on my trampoline while reciting a litany of affirmations. They went something like this:

> I am healthy.
> I am well.
> Illness is no longer a part of my reality.
> Pain is no longer a part of my existence.

> Perfect health is my natural state.
> Perfect health is a choice I make.
> I am in perfect health.
> I love myself.
> I love my body.
> I believe in myself.
> I trust myself.
> I am powerful.
> I am all I need.
> I am who I want to be.
> I am entitled to miracles.
> I am ready and I want one now.
> I know my future is bright and joyous and secure,
> For I am a beloved child of the universe
> And the universe lovingly takes care of me
> Now and forever more.
> Thank you for my perfect health.
> Thank you for my perfect happiness.
> Thank you for my perfect success.

By saying these over and over, I'd convinced myself that they were true. And they became my truth. They became Jim's source of aggravation. (You have no idea how many recitations I could get through in thirty minutes. Your list doesn't have to be this long. In the beginning, I wanted to make sure I'd covered every base. I've since condensed it to the three "Thank yous.")

And then I'd sing "I Love Myself," (song and music by Jai Josefs, Living Love Publications) from Louise Hay's "Loving Yourself" tape, (Meditations, 1984). Try saying this in front of the mirror, looking yourself in the eye. (It gets easier with practice.)

> I love myself the way I am,
> There's nothing I need to change.
> I'll always be the perfect me,
> There's nothing to rearrange.

I'm beautiful and capable
Of being the best me I can.
And I love myself,
Just the way I am.

This stanza was for Jim:

I love you just the way you are,
There's nothing you need to do.
When I feel the love inside myself,
It's easy to love you.
Behind your tears,
Your rage and fears,
I see your shining star.
And I love you
Just the way you are.

Hay's book *You Can Heal Your Life* has been my bible for many years. It offers many practical daily exercises that are inspiring, life-affirming, and short. You don't need to have visited the Holy Land in order to receive benefit. Anybody who picks up this book will be better for it.

A few of her Life lessons you may want to consider and reflect upon:

#25: Everything happens for a reason.
#26: Everything happens when it's supposed to.
#27: Everything is working out for your highest good.

Think about these. Let them inspire hope and help you with acceptance and patience.

When things look their bleakest and you've suffered a setback, reassure yourself with (my) *Lesson #28: If something's been taken away, it means something even more wonderful is around the corner and coming to you.* When friends share bad news and I respond with this lesson, they sometimes call me Pollyanna. But I have found that if you can wade through whatever is weighing you down, a reward awaits you. My friend and financial consultant, Chellie Campbell, says that God has three answers when you ask for something: 1. 'Yes' 2. 'Not now' or 3. 'I have something better planned.'

I changed my view from one of scarcity to one of abundance. *Lesson #29: There are enough babies to go around.* When others conceived, I used to feel like their babies should have been mine. But, of course, they weren't mine. If we believe that babies choose their parents because only those particular parents can provide the lessons needed this time around, then their babies could only come to them. And I figured that mine was somewhere else waiting for me to do something else.

Also on the "Loving Yourself" tape is a moving meditation on abundance and prosperity. You begin by envisioning the ocean. Everyone on the beach has a container to fill from the sea. It can be a teacup, a pitcher, or a vat. But the point is, there is always enough for everyone, regardless of their numbers or the size of their vessels.

I've come to think this way about life. If someone gets the job you wanted, there will be an even better job coming your way. If someone finds the "perfect" guy, it doesn't mean you won't too. There's more than one out there. I believe that there's enough of everything to go around. It helps me to be truly happy for friends' good fortune instead of being wistful about what's lacking in *my* life at any given moment.

The more you give, the more you get. When you help someone, you get it back tenfold. You're not going to run dry. The universe replenishes you. Gerald G. Jampolsky, M.D. writes in *Out of the Darkness Into the Light* (Bantam Books, 1989):

> I think the most important
> Equation in the world is
> That the fullness of one's heart
> Is directly proportional to
> How much love one gives.

It also became important for me to stop judging people. I finally recognized that everyone was doing the best they could. Even when they were not giving me what I wanted, they were doing the best they could do at that moment. (This helped me look at Jim with softer eyes.) If I judged people, I'd invite them to judge me. The Golden Rule about doing unto others comes into play here. Treat others as you want to be treated. And the rule of Karma: What goes around, comes around. Thinking this way allows you to heal childhood hurts, adolescent traumas, and adult mishaps and misadventures. You need to forgive everyone you hold a grudge against, especially yourself.

****

I believe that language is a powerful way to access the mind/body link. It's a way to frame situations and events positively or negatively. The choice is yours. Is the glass half full or half empty? Reframing your language is probably the single most significant change you can make. Think of some common expressions people use that have a very negative message:

> I'm dying for a cigarette.
> I'm sick and tired of that.
> I'm losing my mind.
> I'll do it if it kills me.
> I'll die if that doesn't happen.

Pay attention to what you're saying aloud. Notice the obscenities and negativity in your internal monologue. If you keep telling yourself you're sick, tired, and dying, you will be. Your words create your reality. If a lot of your sentences start with "I can't...," you won't. Focus on what you *can* do. You can record over the old tapes playing in your head. Replace them with new ones that begin with, "I will, I believe, I think I can, I think I can..."

Lesson #30: *Take the word "should" out of your vocabulary.* There are no "shoulds" in life. They only serve as ways to beat up on yourself: "I should be happier," or "I shouldn't be so depressed." You are where you are. You're doing the best you can. Forgive yourself for not being perfect.

I changed my language and stopped shaming myself. I didn't say anything I didn't want to come true. *Lesson #31: Your body hears and believes every word you say.* If I slipped, I'd say "Cancel" (a computer term). I mumble this when I hear friends saying something awful. When they make negative statements, I respond with a low background stream of "Cancel cancel."

When I was really stuck and spooked about all the horrible things that could happen to me, I'd calm myself with the question "What is the real truth?" For example, if you're having thoughts like "I didn't get pregnant again last month. Nothing's working and it never will. I'm going to be miserable and lonely for the rest of my life," ask yourself, "What's the real truth?" My real truth was that I needed to take things one day and one step at a time; that it was probably not a good idea to subject myself to expensive procedures while in this negative mindset. That I didn't know what the future held; that anything was possible. I needed to clear and cleanse my mind of all the junk that had been deposited there by past unhealthy people and experiences and my reactions to them.

In their book *Getting Pregnant When You Thought You Couldn't* (Warner Books, 1993), Helene S. Rosenberg, Ph.D. and Yakov M. Epstein, Ph.D. suggest "Getting Pregnant Self-Talk (GPST)" as a way to clean your mental house.

> Get in touch with my negative self-statements
> Prepare a counterargument
> Say my new statement
> Thank myself

In *Healing and the Mind* Moyers also talked with Jon Kabat-Zinn, Ph.D., founder and Director of the Stress Reduction Clinic at the University of Massachusetts Medical Center and

Associate Professor of Medicine in the Division of Preventative and Behavioral Medicine at the University of Massachusetts Medical School, about the necessity of revamping your psyche. He observed that in situations of great stress, people are not in touch with the current moments of their lives. Because they are too preoccupied with where they want to go and what they want to happen, they are not connected to or living in the present.

The cornerstone of the Stress Reduction Clinic is meditation. This may sound weird to you. I used to think meditation was only practiced by the bald, ankle-belled Hari Krishnas who hand out pamphlets at the airport. Kabat-Zinn demystifies meditation by explaining that it "just has to do with paying attention in a certain way."

Slow, deep breathing is the main engine for proper meditation. Rhythmic breathing allows you to tune out stressors and distractions and focus your wandering mind. I was struck by the ease with which I slipped into a meditative state. It was almost as if my body needed to go there to rest. Apparently this is a common occurrence. Kabat-Zinn says that "People take to our program like ducks to water." I'm convinced humans are wired for this.

Athletes use the meditative state to be completely centered and focused. Think of a diver, a runner, a golfer. The union of mind and body is what allows each of them to excel.

Moyers concluded that while the essence of meditation is not magic, he's still not sure how it works. But, he points out, it's not known how some medicines work, and yet we use them.

One thing is for sure: when you meditate faithfully, you will begin to elicit the "relaxation response" a physical state of deep rest. The relaxation response is the grandfather of modern meditation in this country. The term was coined by Harvard cardiologist Herbert Benson, who reintroduced the centuries-old practice of meditation when he integrated it with conventional medical treatment in his bestseller *The Relaxation Response* (William Morrow & Co. 1975). This mind/body medicine is easily learned, costs nothing, and has no side effects. If regularly elicited, the relaxation response can protect the body from future stress, even when you are not meditating.

The meditative process is user-friendly, and the results can be truly profound. In his book *Brain Longevity* (Warner Books, 1997), Dr. Dharma Singh Khalsa explains, "When you achieve the relaxation response, blood pressure decreases; alpha waves are elicited; oxygen consumption declines; cortisol output decreases, as does muscle tension; immunity is heightened; alertness is increased; and memory is potentiated. Also, blood flow to the brain is increased by up to twenty-five percent."

I know of no substitute for meditation when you are infertile. It's not something you can put off if you are actively trying to get pregnant. You will compromise your efforts to conceive if you don't wind down first. Remember Dr. Alice Domar's success teaching meditative skills to her program attendees. More than half got pregnant once they learned to relax and cope. You can, too. Stop resisting and start breathing.

Many therapists and wise men have counseled that the thing we resist the most is the thing we need to do the most. So I learned to meditate.

Here's how I do it: Sit with a straight spine. Use pillows to make this position comfortable. The alignment is important to keep you grounded on one end and connect you to your higher energy on the other. Switch to diaphragmatic breathing. You'll know you're doing it right by putting your hand on your tummy. It should rise when you inhale and fall when you exhale. Concentrate on your breathing. As you inhale, think: 'Peace;' as you exhale: 'Release.' Or, inhale: 'Help Me;' exhale: 'Thank you.' Or repeat a word or phrase for focus as you breathe in and out. You can pick any word as your focus word or "mantra," like "One, Peace, Lord, etc." (Sasha used to sit in my lap and purr as I did my "Ommmm's.") Let your thoughts move through your mind without judgement. A good start-up schedule is three twenty-minute sessions per week. You may find that you can carve out more time when you start to feel the benefits, like I did.

In his most recent book *The Wellness Book* (Fireside/Simon and Schuster, 1993) with Ellen M. Stewart, R.N., M.S., (who's also on staff at the Mind/Body Medical Institute), Dr. Benson offers his direction to help you achieve the relaxation response.

STOP

TAKE A BREATH
• Release physical tension.

REFLECT
• What is going on here?
• What are my automatic thoughts and exaggerated beliefs?
• Why am I anxious or distressed?
• Am I allowing the problems to get out of perspective?
• Will worrying help? What is the worst that can happen?

CHOOSE
• What can I do? What coping techniques would work here?
• Should I consider my emotional response separately from the practical problem?
• Am I avoiding the best solution because it will be difficult for me?
• What is possible?
• What do I want to do?

It may feel hokey at first. I kept waiting for something momentous to happen. I had trouble shutting out the outside world and often giggled because I felt foolish. When I was in a group, I would sneak peeks at the others to see if I was the only one who wasn't in a trance. But fairly soon, I was able to go into a deep state of relaxation simply by counting backwards from ten. By the time I got to one, I was in la-la land.

As a beginner, a tape can help you become focused. Some that are particularly good at transporting you are Dr. Bernie Siegel's, Louise Hay's, Shakti Gawain's and Marianne Williamson's. These are available at most bookstores. You can also purchase tapes for $10 each by mail from The Mind/Body Medical Institute, Deaconess Hospital, Attn: Tapes, One Deaconess Road, Boston, MA 02215, (617) 632-9525.

A tape is a comforting friend to take to the doctor's office when you undergo inseminations or other more invasive procedures. I had a girlfriend who was a disbeliever. The first time she put on headphones during a procedure, she fell asleep! It's an automatic way to feel centered, grounded, and peaceful no matter what is going on around you. The more you do it, the quicker it will happen for you.

Meditation also enables you to get messages that are vital to your well-being. Meditation allows you to go within yourself and contact your spirit. I believe that we all have a guiding force, an inner voice that resides in each of us. When people say, "I know in my heart of hearts," or "My gut feeling is," or "I know deep down," what they are really talking about is their spirit, their inner wisdom. Most people don't call it that (especially outside of California) but it's true.

When you spend most of your time looking for answers outside yourself, like from your doctor or your mate, you forget to listen to your inner voice, your heart. And that's the real you. When you're so tightly bound to your outside world, you obscure your heart sounds. But if you stop talking and really allow yourself to get quiet, amazing things happen. Frenetic people are out of touch with their inner beings. And when you learn to find calm and enjoyment in your present life, you'll be in more peaceful place to make parenting decisions.

Okay, let's say that you're convinced that this wonderful

person is hiding inside you, but how do you meet her? How do you communicate with her? How do you find out what she (that's YOU) really wants? It takes some practice, but it will become very natural and nourishing.

When you perform meditation, i.e. sitting still, closing your eyes and concentrating on your breathing, you open yourself up for a lot of cosmic communication. Some days I wouldn't get anything. Other times I would marvel at what I'd received.

Sometimes I had trouble tuning out my to-do list. I learned to envision my talking head, put a square around it (like a TV screen) and reduce it in size to a small corner of my entire mental screen. That way, your everyday voice gets to go on but doesn't compete with your solitude. I've found it eventually fades out all together.

On the big inner screen, I would see all things beautiful to me. Foamy waves, warm sand, swishy trees, a rainbow. I could feel the lulling breezes as I sat on a knoll overlooking a beach, surrounded by my favorite flowers: roses, freesia, and tulips. Sometimes I would play music. After a while, the music alone would trigger these scenes, and I would get the same sense of well-being just from the tape.

Pictures of a baby would float by. It was always a girl. I used to see this tiny baby girl dressed in pink corduroy overalls when I first started. But she began to fade, and then I would only see her wrapped in cellophane with a pink bow, like an Easter basket. I longed for her to come back. I felt I was losing her. But another baby girl began to appear. She was a much sharper image. I figured that the first child was the one I lost through the failed adoption. This new one had to be mine.

If you don't think you can find the time for these quieting exercises, you may want to reorder your priorities to make time. I felt fortunate not to have a 9-5 job during most of my infertility. On the other hand, a structured work schedule might have given my brain more respite. I did have obligations, like my free-lance writing assignments, so I wasn't immersed only in my airy-fairy world. I played the corporate wife, entertained and did lots of volunteer work. The latter helped me to keep perspective and allowed me to offer my positive message to others who were starting a lot further back in life than I had.

Meditation is one of the most loving things you can do for yourself, and one of the most positive to reverse your current plight. Another way I tranquilize myself is by reading a meditation from a preferred book into a tape recorder and then playing it back when I want to actually meditate. I found that hearing the instructions in my own voice was most comforting. It was like the public me talking to the private me.

Visualization is a form of meditation during which you play a more active role. Whether you are picturing medicine knocking out an illness or sperm fertilizing your eggs, guiding the embryo safely through your tubes, and nestling it snugly in the lush uterine wall, it's a different kind of mind work.

The difference between meditation and visualization is similar to the difference between non-directed and directed prayer. When meditating, your main goal is relaxation and openness to whatever wisdom is presented. During visualization, you are problem-solving by picturing images of ideal solutions.

In *Love, Medicine and Miracles* Dr. Bernie Siegel describes the advantages of visualization as "Seeing what you want in your mind's eye (and) helping (to) convince your unconscious that it's possible, and that helps create an atmosphere of hope."

I was meditating daily and feeling very powerful. Little miracles began to bolster my faith. Alex broke a toe when he escaped on one of his walks with me. The vet said the toe had to come off because this type of injury never healed properly. I asked for a month to heal it myself. Several times a day, I held his bandaged paw, (which he gnawed on furiously) closed my eyes and imagined green and blue light (green is the color for healing, blue for reducing pain) swirling around his foot. I visualized his foot as perfect and whole. When the bandage came off, his foot appeared fine, but the vet wanted an X-ray. Sure enough, there was no sign of injury. He had been healed.

I wasn't quite so confident in my powers when Jim and I gave our next party. He wanted the dog confined to the garage. I didn't want to ostracize him, but I confess I was afraid to rely solely on white light. Previous party behaviors had included scarfing a huge wheel of Brie, five pounds of cooked and *peeled* shrimp and a giant platter of sushi. So I got mild doggie downers from the vet, but apparently didn't give Alex enough. (I had only wanted him out for the evening, not the summer.) He flopped around all night, banging into guests, garnering sympathy. He didn't eat anything, but I was afraid we'd be reported to the ASPCA.

Jim was having a hard time with my new methodology. He confided to Ben that he didn't buy most of it. "What's all the hocus pocus for?" he'd argue. Ben explained that a lot of the structure was to help beginners get started and relax. "Well, I'm not on the trip rest of you seem to be on and I refuse to feel like a jerk because I'm not." I tried reassurances and cajoling to no avail. He just didn't get it, he didn't want to get it, and that should have been okay with me. It wasn't at first, but then I realized that I could do this part by myself. And I'll admit that some of the practices were even too far out for me. *Lesson #32: You can take what you want and leave the rest.*

One of the most valued parts of my "training" was learning to reframe my life. Envisioning your ideal picture of yourself is a way to project your desires. Picture yourself and your life today. Reflect on that version for a moment. Now replace that mental picture with a perfect version, surrounding yourself with what you want most. (I pictured a perfectly healthy, lupus-free me nursing a tiny, perfectly healthy infant, swaddled in pinks, with Jim besotted at my side.) Frame this new vision in blazing white light. Conjure it up several times a day, when you're brushing teeth, dressing, driving or dishwashing. That way, you are sending a clear message to your higher self and the unseen universe about exactly what you want. *Lesson #33: You MUST remember to ask. Often.*

Many of my "teachers" (friends, authors, etc.) taught me how to create my own inner laboratory, or ideal place for relaxation in my head. I made it my perfect room. A place I would want to revisit time and again. I "decorated" it with chintz fabrics, cushy upholstery, peach marble, gold accents, a fireplace, glass circular walls, extremely flattering lighting, lively classical music, tons of fresh flowers and a view of rocky cliffs and the rolling sea.

Here in my private place I asked for a guide. I believe we all have spirit guides waiting for us to enlist them. During a meditation, I imagined an elevator rising into my lab. I was totally receptive to whomever might appear. When the door opened, I saw him perfectly. I had not made him up. I immediately sensed that he was a completely loving presence.

My guide was very handsome and cavalier, late thirties, longish dark curly hair, wearing a white billowy shirt and black pants tucked into high black boots. He had a deep voice and hearty laugh. (Too bad he was a spirit; I'd have gone out with him in a second.) He told me he would be with me always. And he has been for the last nine years. Whenever I get into a jam or need to feel safe, I ask for Edward's help. And I get it. (He told me his name. I had nothing to do with it.) Sorry if I sound like a flake, but many respected individuals, even august physicians like Dr. Bernie Siegel, report having spirit guides. Dr. Siegel writes of his spirit guide, George, who stands by him while he performs surgery and helps him make hard decisions with patients about their care.

I reasoned that God's got a pretty big job, so Edward helps out when the Almighty's lines are busy. For some of you this may be a stretch. Don't knock it 'til you try it. There's someone waiting for you. (When Jim and I got into an argument, he'd ask, "What's Edward think?" Once, when he was driving me to the hospital for yet another health crisis, I was begging Edward and Norman for relief from the pain. Jim asked, "Norman? Norman? I know about Edward, but who the hell is Norman?")

Since his death in 1990, Norman Cousins has been my writing guide. I never got to meet him; he died just days before an appointment we had scheduled at UCLA. On a subsequent visit to a psychic, I discovered he'd been her client, too. So I had her channel him shortly after his death, and he gave me wonderful insights for the book I'd barely begun to write. He sits with me each day at my computer and guides my hand.

Shakti Gawain's book *Meditations* (New World Library, 1991), offers an exact how-to for creating your inner sanctuary and contacting your inner guide. Just read them into a tape recorder and play them back when you're ready to explore.

After setting up your inner sanctuary, you might want to rearrange your outer bedroom. Feng Shui (pronounced "fung shway") is the 3,000 year-old Chinese art of attracting emotional fulfillment and financial prosperity through object and furniture placement. Having everything in its appropriate place stimulates better loving relationships, fosters good health, and enhances career growth. Some of the wealthiest banks in Hong Kong and throughout the world use Feng Shui. The Feng Shui of the owner or manager's office can affect the fortune of the entire company.

I asked Los Angeles Feng Shui consultant, Marie Garcia, how you could Feng Shui your home environments for fertility. First, some general rules for the bedroom I learned from my interview with her.

• No windows near the head of the bed because of energy losses.

- When you lie in bed you must be able to see the door to the room.
- No mirrors that reflect the bed with you in it. They will amplify and perpetuate the losses and ill health associated with the bed. The mirror sees thought forms and auras and will magnify stress. (Garcia says to cover them with a sheet immediately.)
- No beams over the bed.
- Small fountains of running water in the house bring good luck.

The following ritual comes from *Interior Design with Feng Shui* by Sarah Rossbach, (Arkana/Penguin Books 1991).

The Conceptual Ritual

Take the husband's lunch or dinner bowl without rinsing it and do the following:

Place nine raw lotus seeds and nine dried dates into it
Fill the bowl with water to seventy percent capacity
Expose the bowl to the moon and invite the ling (a type of lunar, prenatal energy) in the universe to enter the house
Reinforce by using the three secrets (see below)
Place the bowl under the bed under the wife's abdomen. The first thing in the morning, for nine days, replace the water in the bowl with fresh water, expose the bowl to the sky and invite the ling from the universe to enter the bowl.

After nine days, pour the water into a houseplant and bury the dates and the seeds into the soil. Place the plant near the front door and perform the three secrets. (See below.)

Repeat (all previous) instructions twice.

The second plant is placed in the living room near the entrance to the room. The third plant is placed in the bedroom in the children's position (creativity area of the bedroom).

Three Secrets Reinforcements
How to Energize the Conceptual Ritual

Body Mudra

Ritual hand gestures to expel, bless, exorcise or calm. One can put one's hands together in prayer at the heart if buddhist gestures are not known.

Speech Mantra

A chant to obtain a proper state of mind. The most common mantra is "om mani pad me hum." Or the heart and mind calming mantra, "gatay boro gatay, boro sun gatay, bodhi swo he."

Mind Visualization

This is an intention, will or prayer in the form of a visualization. Simply visualize the outcome that you want. You can will it or have the intention that it will happen.

"Don't superclean your house," Garcia says emphatically. "The Chinese believe that prenatal energy, called embryonic chi, can't cling to a superclean surface. They need dust particles to cling to. That's why some people that live in immaculate houses can't get pregnant."

There are no limits to your abilities when you tap into your mental prowess, except the ones you put on yourself. Some people claim to have used their mental energy to unclog toilets and repair appliances. I prefer to call a plumber and use my mental resources to effect emotional, spiritual, and physical changes. Since I have no idea how anything works, I wouldn't know what to ask for! (And besides, Jim liked to tinker on weekends. He accused me of picking up the phone whenever something was malfunctioning, regardless of the cost. I found phoning was cheaper in the long run. One electrician told me Jim almost burned the house down "installing" an overhead light.)

After Arizona, I never needed an alarm clock. I'd simply summon my internal timepiece to wake me up by counting backward from ten to one to relax and focus. Then I'd visualize a clock and mentally move the hands to the time I wanted to awaken. I'd tell myself that this was the time I would get up. I haven't used an alarm clock in nine years. (And I don't wake up throughout the night to check the time, either.)

I also surround everything in white light for protection: planes, cars, my body, etc. Then I forget about it and leave the rest to God and Fate. It's about trust. My way isn't the only way, but it works for me and it may work for you.

As an act of faith and to affirm my trust, I bought one baby thing, a book called *Pat the Bunny* that came with a soft, little white rabbit. Laurel bought a baby sweater. We both kept these hidden in our closets, but we knew they were there.

I was given a holy card of St. Gerard, the patron saint of motherhood, by a coworker in New York, and I've carried it with me ever since. The card may be bought at any religious artifacts store connected with a Catholic church.

Another talisman is my Woo-woo doll (from Renee). She's made of cloth, has a limbless body and a shock of straw hair. (To Woo: to seek, to gain, to bring about.) Her tag reads: "The Woo is a benevolent force reappearing to remind us that a positive attitude is essential, that anything IS possible, and as always, peace and love." She's perched on my dresser and I bless myself with her whenever I remember. The doll can be bought for about $45 at any Martin Lawrence Gallery, located in most major malls.

I've also heard that when three people have dreams that you are pregnant, you're getting close. One day Ben called and told me he'd seen me very pregnant in his dreams, dressed in black (my entire wardrobe). Then my Guatemalan cleaning woman managed to communicate that she, too, had dreamt something similar. I was one away.

In *The Conception Mandala: Creative Techniques For Inviting a Child into Your Life* (Destiny Books, 1992), Mark Olsen and Samuel Avital remind us that even though science explains the procreative process in a series of biological events, it is important to recognize that a soul is entering into this plane of existence also. They suggest both partners write separate invitations to the potential child, using their own tone and words.

They use the following as a guide:

1. State your reasons for deciding to invite this child; for example, "We know we have a lot to offer a child;" or "We feel ready to be parents."
2. Express the love and care you already sense for this being.
3. Describe dreams or images that have already surfaced.
4. List what you hope to learn by being a parent.

The authors recommend allowing at least three days to complete your writings before sharing with each other. At that time, they suggest writing together a third invitation that blends the two into a single, unified intent. Then before bed, they advise creating your own ceremony, holding hands and reading the new, fully integrated invitation aloud.

Olsen and Avital feel that speaking the words is important, because it aligns thought with breath and feelings, and plants the invitation in the body as well as the mind. Also, the sensation that you are actually speaking to your (future) child is exhilarating and affirming.

So I started talking to my baby. I knew she was out there somewhere because she had shown herself to me. I welcomed her into my body, into my life, and into my family. (Plus it was very validating to call myself "Mommie." It felt real.)

Mommie is here for you.
Mommie is ready when you are.
Whatever you need to do is okay with me.
Take all the time you need.

I welcome you with all my heart and soul.
I love you unconditionally.
I will always take care of you no matter what.

I began to sense she was near. I would have a fluttery feeling as if I were not alone. Jim thought I needed a straitjacket, but I knew something felt different. When I got my period while all this was happening, I didn't lose faith. I knew that what I *was* feeling *was* real on some level. It felt absolutely tangible. And I could see her often when I allowed myself to relax and drift into meditation.

Many people believe that babies first enter your aura and then enter your body. The authors confirm that once the invitation has been formally presented, you will begin to notice changes. The invited child may appear in your dreams or your daydreams. This is also a good time to listen, because the baby may try to communicate with you. I knew mine was.

(Have you been wondering about all those women who didn't have to write invitations or stand on their heads? The ones that get pregnant at the drop of a hat? Believe me, they have other problems. Infertility just doesn't happen to be their cross to bear this time around. We've all got our stuff. It just takes on different forms in different lives.)

The following interview, from the book *Conscious Conception* (Firestone Publishing and North Atlantic Books, 1986) by Jeannine Parvati Baker and Frederick Baker (segment written by Tamara Slayton), was conducted by Dr. William Kautz at the Stanford Research Institute with a psychic (name unstated) who was part of a research team to determine the optimum conditions for conception and birth.

"Attitude is particularly important at time of conception...The couple must be in agreement, a perfect alignment," claimed the psychic. (We weren't yet, but I figured I'd stay open for us both and when I got the slightest inclination from Jim—ZAP—it would happen.)

Believe it or not, Dr. Stephen Sinatra told me that "When a woman's heart is open, her pelvis will open too." He said that she must be in perfect accord with her husband. He cited several women he knew who had experienced "unexplained" infertility with their first husbands, only to become pregnant easily with their second ones.

The Stanford psychic reassuringly stated that "when a soul has chosen a particular couple and the scene has been set, that it (conception) would occur at the right time."

I took this to mean that our girl had picked us and was waiting for all to be right. That was comforting to me. That way, I felt I was directing my thoughts and love to a specific soul and that she indeed wanted me/us.

The psychic also advised that you yield your will to that of the incoming soul. *Lesson #34: Babies come when they want, not when you want.*

I tried to meditate openly, not on specific subjects, to allow my baby a clear path. You don't want to clog your mind with preconceived ideas of what your baby should be. You must stay open to the "God force" around you. It is crucial that you and your partner explore your spiritual sides. That may be all your baby is waiting for!

Consider this gentle push from best-selling author and mythology scholar Joseph Campbell: "You have to give up the life you planned to find the life that is waiting for you."

CHAPTER VI

LIVE ACTS

"A woman's a woman until the day she dies, but a man's only a man as long as he can." —Moms Mabley

Now that you have yelled, smelled, kelped and elevated your heretofore unconscious brain cells, it's time to turn your attention to the sleeping Adonis lying peacefully at your side.

Lesson #35: Most men need sex to feel loved and most women need love to have sex. Since women also need sex to get pregnant, many will sacrifice closeness for what they perceive to be the higher reward of conceiving a child. Men sense this shift. Sometimes they feel psychologically disconnected from their mates because the woman is focused more on procreating than on pleasuring her man. Separating babymaking from making love can help preserve your marital bond. That's why lots of couples prefer artificial inseminations. Conception then becomes something you do at the doctor's office.

From various sources in the infertility literature, and from infertility survivors themselves, I've gleaned the following suggestions to help couples to overcome the drudgery that sex-on-demand can become.

- Send each other racy, suggestive cards at the office.
- Recall for each other sexy past moments when you couldn't keep your hands off each other.

- Fix dinner together. Make it something you can eat with your hands and feed each other.
- Play with each other under the tablecloth in a restaurant.
- Concentrate on other avenues that don't necessarily lead to intercourse, like bathing together, making out, petting, and oral sex. (The problem with the last one is that the sperm isn't going where it's supposed to. Don't look at it as a wasted ejaculation. Instead, remember a little oral sex goes a long way toward mending fences.)
- Engage in sex play anywhere *but* the bedroom.
- Keep the animals out of the bedroom when it's time for baby sex. (Alex always wanted to join in, licking any body parts that were near the edge of the bed, until we barred him.)
- Reserve one non-work, non-sexual activity per week that you can enjoy together.

The bad memories can overshadow the good times, especially when the good ones are in short supply. But if you focus on why you fell in love and why you initially wanted to be parents together, intimacy can be reestablished and your sex life can be revitalized. Experts and survivors recommend skipping baby sex for a month or two, to lessen your pressure, but caution that lengthy breaks from lovemaking can cause estrangement.

I know many couples who feared their relationships were long lost, and they managed to bounce back. It's normal to feel emotionally drained with little left to give your partner. Hopefully, after the last few chapters, you have learned some ways to replenish yourself. After self-care comes the nurturing of the marriage. It is crucial that you commit yourself to staying emotionally joined to your mate. I have friends who scheduled date nights or weekly meetings to stay connected. They would truly listen to each other without interruption or judgement, so they could both feel heard and understood. These times fostered much-needed affection and good will, which spilled over into their bedrooms.

You may be tantalized to know that scientific research has proven that sexual excitement seems to increase conception rates. (Oh great. Now it has to be exciting? Wait, there's a payoff.) Male fertility rises the second time men have sex in the same day. This is particularly true for those with low sperm counts. In a controlled study, the artificial insemination of rats in one group was followed by their sexual intercourse. Their incidence of conception was almost twice as high as those who were merely inseminated.

Other research supports that the quality of the sexual encounter can influence the probability of conception. In women, sexual arousal creates chemical changes that produce a more hospitable vaginal environment for sperm motility and survival.[1] Therefore, since we know that stress can create a hostile vaginal environment and excitement can create a receptive one in addition to elevating male potency, it will help to keep your sex interesting and fun.

Laurel and her husband are the only couple I know who managed to elude the emotional distancing and heartbreak that so often accompanies prolonged infertility. I remember once when they were meeting for an insemination and her husband arrived late. When she encountered him in the parking lot, he said he just didn't think he could do it. Laurel went with the flow, put aside her disappointment and they enjoyed a quick lunch instead. I totally lack her restraint. If that had been Jim, I'd have run over him with the car. When you're angry at your partner though it's imperative to keep your mouth shut. *Lesson #36: You can always say it later, but you can never take it back.*

This may come as a news flash, but friends have consistently reported that their husbands were more willing to consider their feelings if they (the wives) were employed. The women concluded that because they were sharing the financial burden of the infertility, their men were more open to the process. They believe that even a part time job will help to enhance his respect for you.

It is generally thought that women and men experience infertility differently. Women are more likely to be open about their distress and more open to the notion of therapy. Men often claim that they are not devastated, as their wives seem to be. But many admit to feeling their wife's pain and assume they must be strong for her.

We all know that men on the average are uncomfortable expressing emotions. If the infertility is the man's problem, which it is forty percent of the time, shame and secrecy may shroud the couple. I know from experience that some women even lie and say they are the deficient ones to protect their spouse's fragility. How many men do you know who still brag about "knocking up" their wives? In researching this book, I heard time and again about couples seeking treatment in secret because of the husband's inability to impregnate his wife. More than three million men in the United States are afflicted with this problem. As a society, we need a more accepting attitude and a more solution-oriented mindset.

Beware of interpreting a diagnosis of "varicocele" as a sole cause of infertility. A varicocele is a varicose vein of the testicle normally found in fifteen-twenty percent of men. Once thought to be a major factor in male infertility, it is now controversial at best. Many doctors feel the surgery, varicocelectomy, to correct an underproduction of sperm, is over-performed with inconclusive results. Couples can lose valuable time awaiting a positive surgical result during the six-month post-operative period, when other problems may need attention and could be overlooked. While it is well documented in the medical literature that some men are "cured," there is little explanation for the many more who are not, or for the large numbers with varicocele that father children without having surgery.

Artificial insemination is the first-line, low-tech answer to male infertility. Sperm are washed and selected on the basis of how fast they swim, how strong they look and other factors. Sometimes more than one ejaculate is used to prepare a booster shot in the case of very low counts. If this doesn't work, artificial insemination with donor sperm (AID) is recommended. It is believed that over a half million people are alive today as a result of this procedure. While sperm banks pose an easy physiological and financial answer, their usage creates tricky new problems for the couple.

I would urge you to enlist the help of a therapist before undertaking this course. Some couples I know chose to mix the husband's sperm with the donor's so they could still hold on to the possibility of coproducing their own biological child. While this may work for some, it seems to me that they may not be dealing realistically with all the issues. Coping with the question of their child's identity later on is a very personal, intricate matter. RESOLVE has support groups comprised entirely of couples who have chosen this path and can offer invaluable assistance.

Expect the subject of sperm bank babies to continue grabbing headlines as AID is more widely used and the first generation of children conceived this way demand answers.

So far, there are mostly happy endings. Scientists know that problematic issues fade when the baby is born and the parents begin to bond with their new child. In a follow-up study after eleven years, couples who had used AID reported a high degree of satisfaction. More than ninety-six percent said they would select this approach again. These couples also rated their marriages as consolidated and improved.[2]

It's important to remember that men suffer as much as women during infertility, especially if they are the identified patient. They just suffer differently. Their coping skills in many cases, are mainly denial and silence. Some women assume men don't care because they don't talk. Since coping styles can clash, therapy can help both partners state their feelings in a safe environment and teach them how to communicate to ensure future sharing.

There are now many psychotherapy practices devoted entirely to helping couples navigate through infertility. Either ask your specialist or call RESOLVE for a referral in your area.

Arlene Westley, Ph.D., of Woodland Hills, CA, is one such psychologist. She bottom-lines the biggest hurt and most common puzzle for men: 'She's enough for me. Why aren't I enough for her?' Westley told me that wives have a hard time hearing that message. "If one part of the couple has a lesser desire for a family, they often feel guilty that they don't support their partner or want it quite as much. People must be allowed to not feel congruent on every issue. They just need to be able to hear one another and be gentle and more compassionate toward themselves and their spouses."

A good non-blaming way to approach your spouse with hurts or concerns is to begin with, 'When you said/did _____, I felt _____.' For example, 'When you said you didn't care if we ever got pregnant, I felt afraid that I'd never get a child.' Both of you can get fixed in your positions and create a stalemate. If you accept that *the fear of not getting what you want* is the basic motivator for most volatile exchanges, it will make it easier to alter your behavior so that you can hear and be heard.

Persuasion rarely works in matters of this magnitude. Since forcing the issue often backfires, a moratorium might be advisable. Renee did this with her husband in the beginning of their quest when his knees started to knock. She and I reasoned, 'What's a few months in the whole scheme if it makes him feel like he's more a part of the decision and is coming to it willingly?' It worked. She retreated and asked him to come to her when he was ready. Less than three months later he was raring to go.

I suggest you try reflective listening techniques. When your husband is sounding off, paraphrase his words back to him: 'So what I hear you saying is...,' or validate the feelings underneath the words: 'It sounds like you feel angry, hurt, etc...' When discussions escalate, people are most afraid of not being able to state their position. Agree on a time limit. Set a timer if you have to. That way you know you won't be interrupted when it's your turn, and he knows he only has to listen for a short amount of time. Many of us who have labored long at the negotiating table ultimately found that it's necessary to structure a finite amount of time for infertility discussion. Otherwise you have no relief and it will overtake your marriage.

More sage advice from my circle of friends includes *specifically telling your spouse how he can help you.* Men are fixers, not mind-readers, and they feel helpless watching us suffer. If you're specific, like 'I just want you to hold me while I cry,' or 'I want a foot rub,' or 'I'd just like to be left alone for a few minutes,' you'll get what you need and he'll feel like he's accomplished something. (Speaking of feet, if you have the time, a cheap, under-$10 treat is a pedicure. In the winter, when you have to put on shoes, let your toes dry about twenty minutes, then wrap them in Saran wrap before putting on socks and shoes. When you get home, no smudges.)

There's also the oft-repeated theory of "breakdown before breakthrough." This means you have to hit bottom before you can heal. Looking back, it certainly seems like I was aimed in that direction. I am quite stubborn and did not want to recognize my various problems. I blamed Jim. It was he who was deeply flawed, and it was he who needed electric shock treatments. I honestly could *not* take responsibility for my fifty percent of our troubles. (Sorry, I know this is a tough swallow, but *everything* is 50/50; so start owning up to your half.) I felt if Jim would just fix six things, we'd be fine. He thought the same about me. I also truly believed in my heart that once I got pregnant, our problems would be solved. All I needed was a baby and all troubles would vanish. I was also convinced that once we had a child, Jim would fall desperately in love with it, realize I had been right all along, and we would be transformed and transported to sheer bliss.

What we needed to do was to fix the relationship first. Westley stresses the importance of the marital bond. "The goal of producing a baby is the creation of a family. Hopefully a family that has two healthy emotionally intact human beings at the head of it. When a couple is so eroded by this process, the whole family can become impaired. Preservation and enhancement of the marital relationship is crucial."

If private counseling is unaffordable or not covered by insurance, one way to get some relief and direction is to join a RESOLVE support group. There are hundreds of them nation-wide, they are free (except for annual membership dues of about $50), and full of couples just like you. The groups meet weekly and are centered around a particular issue or focus. For example, you can attend an egg donor group or an in vitro group or an "unexplained" group. For many, finding others with the same problem provides tremendous relief. It is my understanding that the groups are closed, meaning you see the same number of the same faces every week and new people aren't allowed to drift in and out. It's best if you can go together, but better you go by yourself than not at all.

Support groups are not for everyone. My friend Renee attended one and found she was just too agitated to sit and listen to everyone else's problems. (She has since gotten a Master's degree in clinical psychology and is interning to fulfill requirements for her license as a therapist!) If you are extremely anxious or depressed, individual counseling may be a wiser course, like Jim and I chose with my therapist, Lynn. Many therapists will work on a sliding scale.

I, however, still warm a seat in group therapy once a week.

I know it keeps me sane. I can say anything in group and not feel judged. I can reveal my deepest secrets and know they are safe with those seven other women. They cheer me on when I'm on a roll and they help me dust myself off when I've taken a spill. And the group gets in my face if they think I'm off track or I'm furiously trying to justify a questionable move. (I happen to be particularly good at this. My therapist says that I usually have everyone almost convinced most of the time, and I can outlast almost everyone with my arguments until someone spots a hole in my reasoning. But I hang on with my teeth until I'm forced to reconsider my position.) *Lesson #37: Staying stuck is sometimes a lot more comfortable that choosing to change* . If your life isn't working, you may find some wise answers outside yourself. For me, seven heads are better than one.

And these women care for me unconditionally. (The first person that I believed gave me unconditional love was Lynn. I was thirty-four.) I can be scared, sad, mad, or glad, and the group is always there. Sometimes I feel silly after I voice a problem because it never seems that big once I've talked about it. *Lesson #38: Giving your problems air time reduces their hold over you.*

In group therapy, I feel like I'm not alone. That I have a place to go where I can be five years old if that's where I'm at. A place where there is ultimate trust. A place to share hopes and dreams. And when I'm struggling, I can benefit from the experience of others who've faced similar dilemmas and be buoyed by their successes. The love and acceptance is what fosters real growth and healing.

I attribute most of my enlightenment to my weekly sessions with the girls. And a weekly meeting shores you up when you start sagging under the strain of real life. Either I've learned how to avoid most of the land mines or, when I do stumble, I'm not falling as far, so the climb up is shorter and less painful. Just being secure in knowing that I can protect and take care of myself, no matter what happens, frees me up to try new things. *Lesson #39: When all else fails, you always have yourself.*

In learning to let go of the past, I discovered I could forgive others because it was the best thing *I* could do for myself. You don't have to forgive people for the horrendous things they may have done to you, but you forgive them for not being the parent/partner/friend you wanted them to be. Please try to forgive those who have hurt you. I promise you will find it very liberating and healing. Just realize that the healing process takes time.

I've also formed some lasting friendships outside of group with some of the members who have become my surrogate family. The point is, a support group or group therapy can also enrich your life in multiple ways. From sex tips to tennis grips to written scripts for upcoming confrontations, there's nothing that can't be made better by sharing it in a group. Sometimes the thing you're resisting the most is the thing you most need to do right away. So if you're blanching at the thought of baring your soul, you may benefit from a confession session—and soon.

Forgiving someone that's still in your face can be tough when you're not in great shape yourself. Overbearing, "expert," inquisitive, meddling, and otherwise clueless family members need to be given strict limits and boundaries. This is a time to support one another as a couple and take a united stand. Lay out the rules for baby showers, baptisms, reunions, and other sensitive gatherings and stand firm. My advice is not to attend.

Renee had never missed the Jewish holidays in New York with her family. But the year her younger sister, Rose, was five months pregnant, Renee stayed home in Los Angeles. (She conceived that week—I can't believe it would have happened had she been stressed out in New York.) During past Christmas holidays, many of my formerly infertile friends fled to warmer climates where they could escape the family scenes and enjoy themselves anonymously.

If a situation becomes intolerable, say with a parent living in the same town who just won't let up, you may want to propose a joint therapy session. You may think I sound like a therapy-junkie and that it's my solution to everything. For me, it has been tremendously healing, yes. But I'm feeling protective of *you*, and a good way to quiet an irritating parent who's adding to your distress is to have a professional tell them to shut up if they love you!

I can't overemphasize the importance of seeking outside help when you are caught in the infertility quagmire. There's really no downside to therapy, provided you are with a good therapist. You can find one by applying the same procedures that you used to locate and evaluate your medical doctor in Chapter III. I started in individual, moved into couples with Jim, and ended up in group. Most of the time now, I only need be reminded of things I've already learned, because when you're in crisis, you sometimes forget what you already know.

Other benefits of therapy can include helping you improve communication with your doctors, increasing the involvement of the nonsymptomatic partner, or helping you both to know when to say 'when.'[3]

It is quite common for couples seeking admission to fertility clinics to be fearful that if they acknowledge psychological problems, they will be disqualified from the treatment they are so desperate to obtain. As a result, they may conceal considerable degrees of guilt, anger, despair, and helplessness. If the clinic subsequently refers them to a psychotherapist, they often feel singled out as failures and even more distraught and out of control than before.[4]

You don't have to go to therapy for years like I did. I had a host of other issues to deal with besides the infertility. Most doctors believe that brief, focused psychotherapy is the preferred alternative for infertility patients. The goal of such treatment is to strengthen defenses and reduce anxiety.[5]

Every book and research paper I picked up stressed the need for the couple to deal with the feelings of grief and loss that *accompany* infertility before they move on to *resolving* their infertility. And many agree with Westley that working through the grieving process is the most critical work a therapist can do with a couple. She also feels that the length and form of grieving is a very individual matter.

Friends and acquaintances talked to me about grieving over many different aspects of their infertility. One woman bemoaned the fact that this was one thing her father couldn't fix for her. Another is a devout Jew who felt abandoned by her religion. Everyone talked about grieving for the dream of the "perfect little family." Many felt adoption would stop the pain.

Not so, says Marlou Russell, Ph.D., author of "Adoption Wisdom" (Broken Branch Productions, 1996), and an adoptee herself. "People must remember that *adoption is a second choice for all concerned*," she told me. "The losses and gains in adoption are very near to each other."

Westley says that it's not uncommon at all for couples to express, 'This is a very nice baby, but it isn't the baby we really wanted.' Both she and Russell feel strongly that prospective adoptive parents finish grieving for their unborn biological child before undertaking an adoption. Only then can they experience the anticipation and excitement for their coming baby and new family.

One adoptive mother I know well confided that she and her husband *had* to go through the ten years of infertility, the numerous treatments and the subsequent counseling before they could fully accept and appreciate their adopted son and daughter.

"We had to try everything, then we had to let it all go," she says. "Today I can't imagine having any other kids but the ones I've got."

Renee told me this story which allegorically illustrates the challenges of infertility and how you can heal and resolve them.

Imagine you and your husband are packed and prepared for a trip to Australia. You have been saving up and planning to go since you got married. You get to the airport and you are told the flight has been canceled.

The second day, you return to the airport and are told that there's something wrong with the plane.

The third day, you go and are told the flight was over-booked and you have been bumped.

The fourth day, you go and see all your friends getting on the plane but you are told there is no room for you.

A week later, you go back to the airport and see all your friends getting off the plane. They are complaining of jet lag and bad food. You're praying for jet lag.

The next week, you see all your friends getting back on the plane for another trip. Still you are not allowed on the plane.

You and your mate go home and decide there must be another way to get to Australia.

So you hire a boat and go.

In other words, grieving doesn't have to mean giving up. It means giving up your preconceived dream and finding another way to get it. For me, I had to grieve over not being able to make a baby when I wanted to. And my resolution was to hand my dream over to God and accept whatever outcome He wanted for me. For some of you, after the grieving, adoption will be the answer.

You may be cheered by the following good news. Most marriages not only survive the rigors of infertility, they become stronger. Westley told me that in her fifteen years of work, most infertile couples maintained solid love relationships. Although the strain is enormous, she has known very few who've divorced. I find this incredibly encouraging and I hope you take it to heart.

One of the frustrations I fought was trying to explain to Jim just how crushing it felt to be infertile. At the time, I could come up with no analogy that allowed him to really feel my anguish. After many interviews with men, I have tried to portray some events central to a man's existence that would parallel a woman's devastation at not being able to conceive and carry her own child. Here's an exercise that may help your man "get it" at last.

- Look into your memory and imagine yourself as a small, excited boy with your first baseball glove engulfing your hand. Remember how the glove smelled. Remember how big the other kids looked. Picture your dad on the sidelines shouting instructions and encouragements. Remember how badly he wanted you to play little league. Think of how much you wanted to please him. Remember how heavy the bat felt. Feel how frightened you were. Remember how you cried when you didn't make the team.

- Envision being singled out at the amusement park as too small to go on a big ride with all your friends.

- Imagine longing for the fastest bike with all the trimmings, knowing your family's budget could only afford a lesser model. Think about not getting what you wanted, yearning for what the other kids had, and being unable to tell your parents because you were protecting their feelings.

- Envision the science fair, when you entered your home-made project with pride, having observed the rules to work independently. Recall how you were bested by another student whose parent had engineered his slick presentation.

- Remember as a young teen pining for a particular girl, saving up your odd-job money and your courage to ask her out, only to be turned down in favor of a classmate with a bad reputation.

- Visualize applying for your first job, wanting it badly, knowing you were qualified. Imagine replaying the interview a hundred times in your head while you waited for the call, sweating it out, getting the news, losing out. Visualize phoning your parents and telling them of your defeat.

- Suppose you finally find yourself in bed with your dream woman and you ejaculate the moment you feel her body pressed against yours.
- Imagine being fired, with no warning, no severance, no reason.
- Picture coming home from a war in a wheelchair, permanently disabled, to a waiting wife you can no longer make love to or support financially.
- Compare your life to a basket of eggs. Each egg represents a dream. Now consider an imaginary stranger upending your basket. The eggs dive bomb onto the sidewalk. Obliterated.
- Think about enduring each of these incidences consecutively, without much time in between. Try on the feelings of rage, disappointment, shame, impotence, and loss.

What if you couldn't be the hunter and gatherer? Many men told me, "If you can't hunt, you can't be a man." Think about forfeiting your deepest wish. Think of being denied what you were meant to be. Of being passed over for no apparent reason. Of failing repeatedly in front of your loved ones while doing things you were supposed to be good at. Please reflect upon the pain these feelings bring.

Women are meant to be mommies. Our first toys were baby dolls we lugged everywhere, imitating our mothers. Mothering, nurturing, and nesting are as essential to us as breathing. Motherhood is the core of our identity. When that is ripped away, for whatever reason, we don't know who we are. Please try to understand that until this infertility hell is resolved, we feel utterly lost.

CHAPTER VII

ANGEL BABY

"Miracles are natural. When they do not occur, something has gone wrong."
                                    —from the book *A Course in Miracles*

"Miracles never cease."   —Anonymous

You are so ripe!* Ben gushed when he met me for dinner in New York. "You're going to get pregnant if Jim sneezes in your direction. I can feel it!" I felt it too, and had been praying for the best possible outcome to occur.

A few months had passed since the ill-fated adoption incident. Jim had business in New York and I had accompanied him. While he met with clients, I dined out with Ben and Sophia. Jim and I hooked up back at the hotel (the same one in which we'd met), and made wild love. (There's something about hotels that makes me feel randy. Maybe you should try it sometime.)

The next weekend we were home preparing for Jim to leave for a film market in Milan. Before he left on any trip, we would always make love. Things between us were still not entirely peachy, but we both wanted that closeness before being separated for three weeks. I planned to join him in Italy for a week's vacation after he finished working. I knew we needed to discuss his lingering hesitations about having children. "Would waiting another year to have a child be that important to you?"

He looked up at the ceiling while I held my breath. "Well, I guess if you got pregnant now, the baby wouldn't be here for another nine months, and that's almost a year, so I guess that would be okay." I felt like we finally had a shared project. We made love tenderly. I helped him pack. He left for Italy that night.

A couple of weeks later, I began to feel a growing excitement inside. I was certain I felt a new presence, and it wasn't any of my old heavenly buddies. My period hadn't shown up, but since I hadn't been tracking my cycle, I didn't know if it was late. I bought a pregnancy test kit and used it at five o'clock the next morning. I had to wait ten minutes, so I read the directions a hundred times. They read, "If the tip of the test stick has turned any shade of pink, this is a positive result."

I pulled out the stick. The tip was the faintest shade of pink. I held it up eight different ways in the light. I thought I was seeing things. But no, it was PINK! Pale pink, but PINK. I WAS PREGNANT! I fell to my knees and wept. I thanked God and my celestial crew. I sang "Over the Rainbow" at the top of my lungs. And then I quietly welcomed this new little being into mine.

I wanted to tell Jim first, in person, but I wasn't leaving for Italy for five more days. I knew I couldn't possibly keep this news inside me for even five minutes, so I called Ben and Sophia in New York. Ben answered sleepily and I said "Guess what?"

"I already know."

"BEN, I'M PREGNANT!"

"I know you are." (He prided himself on his psychic abilities.)

"I want you guys to be the godparents." He accepted.

I went back to the bathroom to check the stick again. It was still pink. I crawled into bed and talked to my baby until the sun came up. My stick was still pink in the light of day. *I was really pregnant.* I felt so grateful and joyous and special and precious. I hugged myself for hours. My baby had come. And for some strange reason, I was sure it was a boy.

The day before I left for Europe, I had an appointment with Dr. Casanova's office to confirm my pregnancy. As I was driving, I realized it was my brother Robert's birthday. The first one since his death. I thought of a phrase the nuns had taught us, "When God closes a door, He always opens a window." I was looking out the window and I saw a rainbow. I don't know if anyone else saw it, but I did.

A nurse performed my test, which, of course, was positive, and gave me a white plastic square with a plus sign on it that she had used in the test. When I got home, I wrapped it in a Tiffany's box as a present for Jim.

The flight dragged on for an eternity. I had to change planes in London and Frankfurt. I didn't sleep much. I told all the flight attendants I was pregnant. (I felt that was okay because they were strangers.) Jim was waiting at the airport for me with flowers. I kept my mouth shut for the forty-five minute cab ride to the hotel. When we got to our room, I gave him the box. He complained that I had spent money at Tiffany's on something he didn't need (I knew he would). He opened the box and looked at me quizzically.

"What's this?"

"A positive pregnancy test."

"How did this happen?"

"You were there."

He got choked up and we both cried. Then he held me at arm's length and said, "Katie, you're going to be the mother of my child!"

We called our families and close friends and everyone was in happy shock. We went out to dinner with our foreign friends and we told everyone, including all the restaurant help, about our good fortune. When I was asked, I realized I didn't even know when I was due.

Our trip proved to be epically enjoyable except that it drove me crazy that I couldn't drink any of the legendary Italian wines I was offered. I felt a little tired, but the Italian countryside always revived me. We got home and celebrated my thirty-sixth birthday. I was looking forward to my first obstetrical visit with Dr. Casanova the following week.

I read every baby magazine in the waiting room before I saw him. Part of me still couldn't believe I was pregnant and yet I felt it inside. I felt contented and wildly thrilled at the same time. I never considered for a moment that anything could go wrong. I knew God wouldn't take from me what He had given me at last.

Dr. Casanova tore into the exam room. "How did this happen? You didn't have the tubal surgery I told you to have. I haven't seen you in months." His eyes burned with anger. I felt taken aback by his rage. It seemed as if my becoming pregnant had challenged his medical authority.

I wanted to explain my recovery to him. He insisted on examining me first. As he dragged the ultrasound machine toward me he said, "Let's see if we even get a heartbeat."

I should have gotten up then and left, but I wanted to prove him wrong. Sure enough, there was a heartbeat. It was the tiniest flutter—like Tinkerbell—but strong and sure. As I felt the rush of emotion roll over me, he began lowering the boom.

"Okay, you're thirty-six. You're going to have an amnio. You have lupus, so you're going to have to take drugs. I'll have to take the baby early—I don't know how early—it's going to be touch and go."

I bolted upright from the table and cut him off. I told him I'd gotten the lupus into remission, so there was no need for panic. I tried to tell him how, but he would hear none of it. Then I got mad and told him I was going to do this *my* way. He exploded. "You could die, your baby could die, and if I were your husband, I'd divorce you immediately!" I flew out of his office, badly shaken, but I knew I was healthy and so was my baby. That was the last time I ever saw him.

I was now two months pregnant, with no doctor, and Jim was nervous. But I remained calm as I began my search for a good OB. I wanted a doctor that would be sensitive to my needs. (What I really wanted was a home birth, but Jim keeled over when I told him this.) I was considered a high-risk patient because of my medical history, even though my physical and mental picture had changed dramatically. After all, by God, I had gotten pregnant. I wanted a doctor who would treat me with respect and acknowledge that, yes, I had improved my health, and thus the pregnancy.

I had been doing volunteer work at UCLA and was told about a Dr. Khalil Tabsh, who was at the time Chief of Obstetrics there. He sounded awfully medical to me, and I was just fine, thank you, and having a normal, healthy time of it. But friends urged me to seek him out. Since Tabsh only took on sick women, I had to have an influential friend call and get me an appointment. I was almost three months along by this time.

If Dr. Casanova hadn't been such a maniac, I might have stayed with him and missed meeting one of the most remarkable medicine men of our time. Tabsh was in his early forties, tall, slim, handsome, and warm. I grilled him for thirty minutes before I would let him touch me. All of his nurses called him K and he said I could too. (No one could pronounce Khalil correctly.) I told him my story and he listened attentively. I told him how I had engineered my recovery and he cheered my victory. I felt respected by a doctor for the first time in my life. He told me he would accept me as a patient under one condition: If complications arose, I would agree to whatever treatment he considered necessary. I said yes and the deal was struck. K said I'd be the only healthy one in his practice. "This will be fun," he said with a twinkle. I was in heaven.

Jim felt relieved because I now had excellent medical care;

I felt satisfied that a doctor had finally taken me seriously. I had an impending decision about whether or not to undergo am-niocentesis and K had wisely left it up to me.

I was not happy about having this test. I felt certain my boy baby was perfect, and besides, I was willing to accept whatever God had sent. Jim went ballistic when I suggested bypassing the procedure, so we ended up back in therapy. Lynn helped me to reframe the amnio as something I could do for Jim. A present to give him. When I looked at it that way, I felt okay about cooperating. I was seventeen weeks pregnant when I had the test.

K located the baby on the ultrasound screen and asked if we wanted to know the sex. We did and he said, "It's a koukla!" (The Greek word for "little doll.") Tears streamed down my cheeks. "Oh no. Are you sure? What's that?" Jim asked as he pointed to a long wavy line on the monitor. "It's the umbilical cord," smiled K.

On the way home Jim slumped in a mild funk, explaining that he thought for the last four months he was getting a son, and it would take him some time to digest our news. (I sure was glad we hadn't waited to be surprised in the delivery room.) I think I had believed it was a boy because I wanted one for him. But 'it' was a 'she,' and I was ecstatic. It was my baby girl that I had seen so many times during meditation, and she was on her way.

Jim lightened up by the time we got home, joking about gunning down suitors and footing college *and* wedding ex-penses. I could tell he was disappointed, so to comfort him, I said, "We can have a boy next time." He paled as a look of sheer terror filled his eyes.

We got good news from the amnio results. Then K sent me to a pediatric specialist for a sonogram of the baby's heart. He said it was routine and I didn't question him. This other doctor, however, felt it was his duty to fill me in. As I lay there uncomfortably on my back for a solid hour, he ominously reported that lupus mothers have a twenty-five percent chance of having babies with heart problems. Something about complications in the electromagnetic field. But, he assured me, "A pacemaker can be inserted around age twelve and the child can live a pretty normal life." I wanted to strangle him. For the remainder of the hour, I repeated affirmations out loud, convincing myself that she was completely healthy. And she was. Her little heart was perfect. I looked at it as another test of my faith. God, however, was not finished with me yet.

At the beginning of my fifth month, the lupus attacked with a vengeance. I hid the pain of my aching joints from K and Jim for over a week. When I finally told Jim, he begged me to call K. I was still in denial. I couldn't believe the lupus was back. I believed I had conquered it. I couldn't admit failure. I could do this alone. I had done it before.

Jim pleaded with me. He said it was one thing to gamble with my own body, but I had to think about the baby's. She could be at risk. I was twisted in knots. I saw K the next day and cut a deal with him. I would go to Arizona for the weekend. If I was no better when I returned, I would go on medication to halt the onslaught of the disease. It was picking up speed and the longer it went unchecked, the more danger I was in.

There was no magic for me in Arizona this time. The excruciating pain cut through all my defenses. I felt as if my body had been taken over by aliens. I stayed in bed most of the weekend, unable to participate in the activities, chanting affirmations and begging God for help. I could neither believe nor accept the idea that I could not will myself well. The assembled group was praying for me. Being prayed for is really scary. I felt like a lost cause.

I returned to LA feeling minimally better, so I insisted on driving myself, alone, to K's the next day. I kept up a good front and asked that he give me just a few more days before prescribing drugs. Part of my resistance stemmed from denial, but another part involved the drugs themselves. Steroids are the treatment for acute lupus. These are powerful drugs with major side effects—only for me, not the baby. But her shelter was falling apart and she needed a safe haven until she was ready to emerge. I kept praying for God to wave His wand.

Two nights later, while Jim attended a business dinner, I discovered I could no longer walk. I crawled into the bathroom on my knees and hoisted myself onto the toilet. Then I couldn't get off. So I fell off and crawled back, sobbing and defeated. I called K and he said he would phone in his orders to the emergency room. I left Jim a note and called a neighbor, who carried me to the car. I felt racked with guilt for having compromised my baby's welfare. I felt God had deserted me. The lupus raged inside me like wildfire. It felt scarier and more destructive than ever before.

By the time Jim got my note and called the hospital I was heavily dosed with steroids and ready to leave. When the neighbor dropped me at home, I told him Jim would get me up the stairs to our bedroom. I called and called to Jim, but it was late, he had fallen asleep, and he never heard me. So I dragged myself and my belly agonizingly up the two flights, feeling utterly abandoned.

I had refused pain medication because it could cross the placenta. The steroids didn't work right away, so relief came slowly. Then I started to feel racy, jittery, like I'd just downed ten espressos, and I couldn't sleep more than a few hours at a time. More side effects began to appear in the following weeks. Dark facial hair and acne complimented my moon-sized face, while the hair on my head started thinning. Because of the lupus, my eyes and lips swelled up like a prizefighter's. I'd look in the mirror and not know who was in there. But I felt the disease was loosening its grip, and the baby appeared to be well in the countless ultrasounds K performed to keep tabs on her.

Jim and I started talking about names. In Greek culture, first-born children are named after their (Greek) grandparent of the same sex. Luckily, my mother-in-law was named Mary, not Aphrodite. I wanted Rose for her middle name, after the rose crystal and my maternal grandmother, but I couldn't imagine calling her Mary. In Catholic school, all the nuns had Mary in their names as did most of the girls in my class. So while I was meditating I asked my baby what she wanted to be nicknamed. Moments later letters floated by: M-i-m-i. It was perfect.

Jim liked it too, and so she became Mimi Rose.

In my sixth month, Ben and Sophia invited me to a three-day conference in San Francisco, featuring an Irish healer. His name was Finnbar and he was the seventh son of a seventh son, which according to Irish legend, gave him supernatural healing powers. Although I thought his name was goofy and his price tag exorbitant, I was game for any kind of healing. The combined cost for the airfare, hotel and weekend seminar totalled a shocking $900, so Jim naturally hesitated about my going. I talked him into it, got K's blessing, and promised them both not to flush my drugs down the toilet while I was there.

Finnbar's success rate was about fifty percent, and he admitted he had no idea when or whom he could heal. I couldn't wait for him to get his hands on me. He said a cure usually took the laying on of hands three times. I made sure I was at the front of the line each day.

I never expected to come home from a healing seminar in a wheelchair, but I needed one to deplane. Jim was beside himself when he saw me. I explained that Finnbar had said people who receive "the cure" often get worse before they get better. Jim made a scene in the terminal because he felt so concerned about me and the baby. I almost couldn't blame him.

About this time, K conducted an internal exam and discovered I had an incompetent cervix, probably caused by the wear and tear of previous surgeries. He told me I could not have sex for the remainder of the pregnancy. I laughed; Jim had been afraid to have sex since we'd conceived.

In the meantime, my feet had started to grow. No one had told me that this was a side effect of pregnancy. I went up two shoe sizes, which necessitated buying "sensible" flats. I felt like Bigfoot. (I never did get back to my pre-pregnant size seven. I stayed a seven-and-a-half, which meant I had to buy *all* new shoes. I guess there are worse things in life!)

Two weeks later, an ultrasound revealed that I had placenta previa. My placenta had partially dislodged from the uterine wall and was hovering dangerously close to my cervix. K ordered modified bedrest, again for the duration. I could walk around the house and drive to his office once a week, but that was it. He also informed me that this condition ruled out a vaginal birth which had always been part of my fantasy. I felt great disappointment over this loss.

Part of me felt deeply angry that my body was so fragile and imperilled. What had I done wrong? Dr. Rx had warned that fifteen percent of lupus mothers have flares during their second trimester, but I had dismissed this the moment I heard it. Not for me. I was well.

Throughout all these trials, I continued to instinctively feel that Mimi was thriving. I experienced her as a sweet, peaceful presence within me. While I truly never worried about her, I felt enraged and frightened for myself. I knew there had to be a reason behind all of my health complications. I obviously had more lessons to learn, but I couldn't figure out what they were.

I ventured that the reasons would reveal themselves to me in the fullness of time. I consoled myself with the fact that I was, after all, very pregnant with a healthy baby, which tests continued to confirm, and that she would be in my arms very soon.

As you may already know, a major side effect of taking steroids is weight gain. At thirty weeks, I had only gained eighteen pounds. (Jim had gained twenty.) K and Dr. Rx were amazed that I hadn't blimped out. They checked my thyroid and all was well, so K ordered a glucose tolerance test. It turned out that I had gestational diabetes, a common response to the amount of drugs I was taking. I was hospitalized for a week to stabilize. When I was wheeled onto the floor and saw the huge MATERNITY sign, I couldn't believe I was actually there. What a thrill, and what a reality check.

Jim was in Australia and offered to come home. I told him there wasn't much he could do to help, and to finish his business trip. By now I felt confident going it alone.

After a week, the doctors informed me that the diabetes was only temporary. The bad news included the fact that I had to give myself two insulin shots daily in the thigh and take my own blood by pricking my finger every four hours. The results had to be phoned in around the clock. But I was still pregnant and I felt I could endure anything. After losing four pounds in the hospital, I finally started to put on some weight. (My final weight gain was twenty-two pounds. Jim's was twenty-four.)

As I limped toward the finish, I hit one more bump. Actually there were about seven of them. Hemorrhoids, that is. I had to sit on an inflatable donut until the end. (And they took their sweet time going away after my delivery. Even the anesthesiologist commented on "the whole family back here," when he was inserting the epidural in my spine before the delivery. Imagine my mortification.)

Around this time, Jim started to get shaky about his impending fatherhood. He told me he didn't feel ready. I pointed out that this time it wasn't up to him. We were living according to Mimi's timetable.

At thirty-three weeks, my friends threw me a baby shower, the first one I'd been to in almost four years because of my infertility. I got some wonderful frilly outfits for the baby and lots of sterling silver. (The bare necessities.) Over thirty women were there, most of whom I hadn't seen in months because I'd been so ill. I relished every moment of their caring support and positive energy.

That night the pains started. I felt like I was being slammed up against a wall. Jim and I got out the books, timed the contractions, which came irregularly, and determined this was false labor. It was too soon for the real thing. To sidetrack me, he kept ducking under the covers to talk to my stomach.

"Hello Mimi. This is Daddy. Do you want to come out and play? I'll buy you dollies and give you horsey rides." I never loved him more than at that moment. He helped me through the night.

The next day, K confirmed the worst. I was having pre-term labor. And the labor was causing the lupus to sneak up on me again. Mimi was doing fine, but I was falling apart. He had to increase my steroid dosage. One positive residual of the steroids is that they help the baby grow quicker by allowing her lungs to mature faster. Also, according to K, girls typically mature faster than boys, and diabetic mothers usually have heavier babies. (Just think, I had all that going in my favor!) Perhaps Mimi knew her time inside was running out and she was preparing to be born. K wanted to get her to thirty-four weeks, which is the earliest gestational time when she could assuredly breathe on her own. (A full term pregnancy is forty weeks.) He prescribed more drugs to halt the labor. Although they were effective, they made me feel like I'd drunk twenty cups of coffee a day.

My mood improved somewhat with the delivery of the white Italian lacquer baby furniture, purchased by my in-laws. (Mimi was the first grandchild.) I exhausted myself moving furniture and decorating the nursery. After I finished, I sat in the rocking chair and savored the baby's surroundings, all pink and new. What a relief to be nesting at last.

My nursery exertions triggered the return of the contractions. The stress of my many complications sparked a panic attack which exacerbated the pain from the lupus. The steroids and other drugs made me feel speedy and paranoid. It took all my courage to stay steady while performing my daily blood sample rituals. I prayed for my hanging placenta, my loose cervix, and my contracting uterus to stay strong so that I could reach the thirty-four-week mark.

I felt like a race car driver careening on the shoulder with just three tires. I was barely thirty-four weeks when K performed another amnio to determine if Mimi's lungs were ready. They were, and he scheduled me for delivery the next afternoon.

I watched the clock all night, and during the wee hours I meditated on my dream that was about to come true. "I'm having a baby today," I thought. I felt a mixture of awe, relief and anxiety.

When we arrived at the hospital, there was no room ready for me, so I camped out in a curtained holding area. Jim crawled in bed with me and we both fell asleep.

At seven o'clock that night, K arrived and gave the orders to have me prepped for a C-section. Fifteen minutes later, he burst in and said he had an emergency that he had to deliver before me. I later learned from K that if the operating room hadn't been readied for me, he might not have been able to save the other woman and her baby. I felt thankful that my impending delivery had helped rescue another mother and child from danger. This vital connection to the miracle of life put me in a philosophical mood as I waited my turn.

At nine o'clock, the anesthesiologist and nursing staff descended upon me. They wheeled me into the operating room and administered the epidural. I was prepped, strapped down and hooked up to the monitors. Then I broke down in tears. The weight of the last eight months came crashing down on me and I couldn't be brave for a minute more. My emotions ran riot.

Jim was summoned before I was fully draped and got a great view of me beached on the OR table. Although I didn't see him approach, when he slid his hand in mine, I felt instantly comforted. Our camera picked that moment to fail us, so K himself left in search of a Polaroid. A Mozart piece that I had played throughout my pregnancy filled the room. K returned triumphant and asked if I was ready. I yelled "Yes!" over the music.

****

As I pored over Mimi's first pictures in the recovery room, I realized something which astounded me. I was born twelve years, twelve days and twelve hours before my brother Robert. My birthday is on the twelvth of the month. Mimi was born twelve months, twelve days and twelve hours after Robert died. Her birthday is also on the twelvth of the month. I knew Robert had something to do with this magical occurrence, and I felt very grateful to him.

****

I came home from the hospital without my baby, another dream dashed. I ached for her. The first time I saw her after delivering, her black curls had been almost completely shaved off in order to insert an IV into her head. Imagine the trauma I felt. She was hooked up to monitors because she had sleep apnea, or breathing abnormalities. The doctors refused to discharge her and I felt quite helpless.

I breastfed her in the hospital and pumped my milk when I was home. I put a cloth diaper dampened with my breast milk in her isolette so she could smell her Mommie. This was a harrowing time. I felt like a ghost in my own life because she wasn't home where she belonged. After all I'd survived, there still was no baby in the crib. I made Jim call the NICU every four hours to check on her. I was a postpartum mess, but he anchored me to reality and I clung to him.

After ten days we brought her home. I insisted on being wheeled out with her in my arms for the video camera, just like the regular mothers. Thirty-six hours after her homecoming, I found blood in her diaper. I called her doctors and they referred us to Drs. Frank Sinatra and Danny Thomas (yes, these are their real names) who were pediatric gastroenterologists at Childrens' Hospital.

Mimi looked so small on their exam table. I held her down as they examined her and drew blood. I was consumed by fear and a sense of helplessness. As she cried, my breasts leaked. They determined that she had a lactose intolerance and told me to change my diet from cow's milk to soy milk. It worked and she was fully recovered in two days.

Because she was a preemie, she had to be fed every two to three hours. I was producing a quart of milk a day, getting virtually no sleep, and fighting the lupus with all my strength. (I did manage to slip out to the beauty salon for a perm when Mimi was five weeks old. I mean, I wasn't dead, I was just sick and tired.)

I felt no anger at my body anymore, for it had produced this exquisite little creature. My anger at God had abated because I'd obviously gotten His help, too. But I couldn't find a reason for my continued physical suffering and it confounded me.

There were days when my hands and arms hurt so much I couldn't lift my baby out of her crib. I felt so guilty for failing her this way. So we hired a nanny, who didn't come cheap, and Jim's worst nightmare came true. I'd had a baby and was too sick to care for her myself. I felt my husband beginning to slip away.

I knew that new babies, especially first ones, could upset the balance of a marriage. But I was determined that we'd weather this initial phase, my health would improve and our family would thrive.

After my six week check-up, we went out for dinner to

celebrate and I was looking forward to resuming our sex life, even though it felt a little scary. After our date, we were both so tired, we crawled into bed and fell fast asleep. This became our pattern, unfortunately, a rut from which we never fully emerged.

****

While I was enraptured by my child, Jim seemed to be detaching emotionally from both of us. I wanted the guy who'd been so strong those first weeks of her life to come back to me. It was as if an angel had inhabited his body then and had suddenly taken flight. I visited my therapist, discouraged and disappointed, and she reasoned that Jim had been able to rise and shine for a short time, and he had simply reverted to his standard behavior. I knew he was capable of heroics, and more than anything else I wanted him to enjoy our new life together as a family.

As much as I desired the protective new Jim, he wanted the carefree old Kate. I think he felt jilted, for I'd fallen in love with someone else: Mimi. Jim wanted me to reenter our former social whirl and I could barely go to the bathroom unassisted. He often paced like a caged animal at home and needed to be around adults who could talk about something besides babies.

I began to encourage him to go out without me. I tried to join him when I could, but I just couldn't keep up physically. His business travel increased, and although I felt awfully lonely at first, the distance brought me space and peace.

In the meantime, the animals were holding their own. Sasha the Siamese couldn't understand why he couldn't flop on top of Mimi while I nursed her. He took to sleeping in her crib for those first months while she occupied the bassinet in our room. Alex exhibited deep jealousy, but he stopped growling at her after a couple of months. He sensed his position had been usurped, but he tried to make the best of it, allowing me to prop Mimi up against him for photo ops.

I finally had my girl, bless her heart, but my body felt like it was in ruins and my marriage seemed doomed. I felt completely overwhelmed. I could barely take care of myself, let alone Mimi and Jim. My therapist Lynn told me I had to put myself first or I wouldn't be any good to either of them.

I knew that neither one of us was getting our needs met, which brewed mutual resentment. Jim felt that I had gotten the baby I wanted, and he had lost me to her and to the lupus again. Plus, the full-time nanny was costing him a fortune, which he didn't take lightly. "What about me?" became the recurrent refrain in most of our conversations.

Being a world-class rebounder, however, I was determined to heal my body, resurrect my marriage, and become the best Mom in the world. I convinced myself that all I needed was some sleep.

****

Much to my sorrow, I couldn't cheerlead myself or Jim out of our problems. Although we went for joint counseling for almost a year and a half, we found ourselves unable to reach any kind of resolution. I moved out with Mimi when she was nineteen months old. Even though my body was weak, my spirit felt strong, and I carved out a new life for us one day at a time.

Now that I had my precious child, I found myself providing moral support for my girlfriends and for other women, referred to me by my doctors, who struggled through their own sagas of infertility. It felt hugely rewarding to play "big sister" to women whose plights so resembled my own history. I also felt I had a mission to facilitate the arrival of the many little souls trying to find their paths here. In the next chapter, I recount some of the dramas in which I played a role, as well as some inspiring stories I've collected along the way.

CHAPTER VIII

MORE JOY

"Come to the edge, he said
They said: We are afraid
Come to the edge, he said
They came.
He pushed them...
and they flew."

—Guillaume Apollinaire

If my melodrama grabbed you by the throat, wait until you hear about Laurel's.

Laurel's doctor quickly diagnosed that their infertility problem lay with her husband, Mark. He had a varicocelectomy, and his sperm count increased considerably. Since it was still on the low side, her doctor used the sperm washing method before inseminating her. After many tries, she became pregnant while I was carrying Mimi.

We interpreted this as divine intervention, since she and I had both been diagnosed with lupus by Dr. Rx, one week apart the previous year. Our husbands also worked together and had been friends for many years before meeting us within the same month. Neither of us had sisters. We're both third generation Irish from Galway with lots of brothers. We're not twins: I have thicker hair, she has a skinnier body. She's loved one man in fifteen years, I've lost count. But we are as close as sisters. Unlike me, however, the lupus hit her much earlier in her pregnancy and to her great sorrow, she miscarried at eight weeks.

The next year proved a long one for both of us. One weekend we were attending a sales conference in the wine country in Northern California with our husbands. Mimi was ten weeks old, and I experienced a serious relapse. Laurel immediately took charge. She phoned Dr. Rx and got a referral to a physician in San Francisco. Then she rented a car and drove me sixty miles to his office. Although he put me on a much heavier dose of steroids and I was devastated by this setback, when Laurel reminded me that at least I'd gotten my little girl, I thanked heaven for my good fortune.

A year later, Laurel became pregnant for the second time via artificial insemination and Pergonal. Since her lupus had been quiet for many months, her body was medication-free.

Eight weeks into her pregnancy, her husband found her on the bathroom floor, ghost-white and writhing in ferocious pain. Dr. Tabsh rushed to meet them at the hospital.

He took one look at her and surmised she was bleeding internally. The ultrasound showed him that she had conceived twins. While one lay in her uterus, the other lay trapped in her right tube. Tabsh intervened immediately, removing the ectopic pregnancy and saving the fetus in Laurel's womb. Since she had undergone major abdominal surgery, she was confined to hospital and home for weeks. The stress from the operation triggered lupus symptoms and Tabsh prescribed steroids.

At eighteen weeks, Tabsh performed another ultrasound and looked grave. He asked Laurel and her husband to meet him in his office. There he explained that the baby, a boy, was "not progressing uniformly." His head looked normal, but one femur was only nine weeks along. Because the boy's health could not be improved, and because her continuing pregnancy could irreparably damage her fragile state of fertility, Tabsh recommended a "D&E" (dilation and extraction) to terminate the pregnancy. Laurel was referred to a caring, compassionate doctor and staff. She underwent the procedure at nineteen weeks. It nearly ruined her emotionally.

It's hard not to ask 'Why me?' when mourning this kind of loss. But she and her husband found comfort in each other. Laurel's fertility doctor observed that at least they were conceiving and could try again.

Laurel continued with great bravery and conceived again, one year to the day of the D&E, using Pergonal and insemination.

Tabsh found twins again, a boy and a girl, and they were both in the right place. Only this time Tabsh took an extra precaution. He had Laurel give herself two shots a day of Heparin, a blood thinner, to prevent clotting in the uterus.

A few weeks later, her labwork looked suspicious, so Tabsh increased her steroids. These so suppressed her immune system that she developed a vicious case of shingles on her head and right side of her face. (She had to miss my thirty-ninth black tie birthday party. We decided a wide-brimmed hat just wouldn't do the trick.) Cautious optimism followed, and I prayed for the health of the mother and her babies.

An ultrasound at eighteen weeks showed the little girl was small. Although the baby boy looked robust, Tabsh could do nothing for the girl without jeopardizing the boy. Each week, they watched with anguish as she continued to deteriorate. They finally said goodbye to her at twenty-six weeks. This forlorn little girl was the fourth baby they had lost.

There was no way for Tabsh to remove the little girl's lifeless body without endangering the healthy boy, so Laurel was forced to carry her the remaining ten weeks. She and her husband worried that their joy at the moment of their son's birth would turn to despair during the delivery of the baby girl's remains.

Poor Laurel and Mark never knew the elation that a positive

pregnancy test usually brings. For them, the news meant marshalling all their emotional resources to prepare for the possible onslaught that could lay ahead. It's not that they harbored negative thoughts, but fighting the fear and staying calm became a full-time job.

Laurel lit candles on the anniversaries of the "deaths" of her little beings. We talked often and for hours. She would ask me to repeat over and over my own lessons about hope, tenacity, faith and trust, which I finally put on tape at her request. When she felt like drowning, she was comforted by hearing, 'I know your baby is coming to you,' and 'If I could do it, so can you' playing throughout her house. She said my message gave her inspiration and reassurance. We talked even then about my writing a book to help other women get pregnant and stay pregnant.

I marveled at the durability of Laurel and Mark's marriage. As their boat was rocked time and again, I watched as they gripped each other even harder. Tragedy had torn Jim and me apart, but it seemed to cement Laurel and Mark together. She confided that they were still enjoying sexual play, even though it was somewhat limited and called for some improvising, up until the end of this last pregnancy.

I attended Laurel and Mark's long-awaited baby shower, with this poem I'd written and framed as my gift.

ONCE UPON A TIME
The path was fraught with twists and turns
And filled with lessons to be learned
A wish to be fulfilled in June
Then the dish ran away with the spoon.
Beyond the beyond became the call
When reality made no sense at all
And dreams were dashed like bursting balloons
Could cows jump over the moon?
A baby girl's light burns forever bright

Like a winking star on a moonlit night
A quartet of angels, a heavenly tune
Serenade jumpers over the moon.
A leap of faith, a lonely jump
A last sum of courage over the hump
A little boy's laughter resounding soon
And the cow jumped over the moon!

After Mark read the poem aloud, Laurel asked me if I knew that she had themed the decor of the baby's room based on the cow and the moon nursery rhyme. I'd had no idea. The poem had poured out of me spontaneously. Just another serendipitous event in our lives.

Tabsh conducted another amnio at thirty-six weeks and found the baby boy's lungs were mature. Laurel was two centimeters dilated so the decision was made to induce labor. Her body had already begun labor on its own and Tabsh wanted to avoid a C-section with a long recuperative period. After thirteen hours of hard labor, a blood pressure monitor revealed that Laurel was "in distress." Tabsh and his nurses raced down the hall to the OR pushing her gurney with Mark running at her side.

Eric was born weighing six pounds, one-half ounce, safe and sound. As it turned out, a lot of the female fetus had atrophied and the tissue had been absorbed by Laurel's body. What remained was delivered along with the placenta, masterfully handled by Tabsh. The joy of Eric's birth was not compromised in any way.

Tabsh had suspected all along that the lupus had nothing to do with the baby girl's demise. The pathology report later confirmed this, and stated that there had been a "true knot" in her umbilical cord.

Laurel got to take Eric home with her, ironically on the same day I had taken Mimi home three years earlier. Another one of our "coincidences." Laurel was just shy of her forty-first birthday when she became a mom. She felt immensely grateful and relieved that Eric was finally here. He, like Mimi, was a sweet, peaceful being. She and I joked that after all we'd endured, God had had the courtesy to send us angelic babies.

Laurel and I share a fellowship of pain. When I would get ominous bloodwork, she understood, without preamble, what it meant. After Eric was born, I developed a case of urticarial vasculitis, which produced horribly itchy lesions all over my body. I had to be rushed to the emergency room during the L.A. riots after curfew. I'd been on a low dose of steroids and had to bump way up again. She followed my drama with a case of Bell's palsy, which numbed and paralyzed half of her face, as if she'd had a stroke. Again, hers had nothing to do with lupus. The treatment? Huge doses of steroids. We compared bullfrog faces. Our humor bordered on gallows as only two people who have endured similar indignities can understand. We both know what it's like to go to hell and come back.

Laurel characterizes our illnesses this way: mine is chronic, hers is acute. Hers only went on the warpath when she was pregnant, mine kept showing up for unscheduled appearances. She is now practically in remission—she takes minimal medication and she is symptomless. Mine is contained, with occasional eruptions, by lots of medication. Although I've had a longer time with active lupus, hers has been more trouble-laden and complicated.

We both found it impossible to meditate on steroids. It's hard to quiet your mind when your heart is thumping, your pulse is racing, and your blood is pounding in your ears. One remedy we used to combat the steroid assault was the shower. We would just sit on the floor and let the hot water beat down until it ran out.

We kept journals religiously until our dedication dried up.

"I'm sick of this personal growth stuff," she once told me. I had to agree: physical torment saps the spirit.

When you've looked death in the face, as I have for myself and she has for her would-be children, your perspective is profoundly altered; your priorities forever changed. I wouldn't be here today without Laurel's help. She has been my teacher, my sister, my friend-in-grief. She helped me find hope in my bleakest moments.

I remember the many desolate times we shared—how we'd call each other—surprise!—from the hospital. Conversations began with, "Don't be alarmed, but I'm in..." We've both had so many physical and emotional trials in addition to the lupus. And yet, haunted as we are, with heavy losses and high body counts, we love life and live it to the fullest with true joy in our hearts. I largely attribute this to the fact that we have always loved and supported each other unconditionally. We always will.

When Eric was about three, Laurel casually called me with another dramatic announcement. She was pregnant again. This time, it happened at home, without inseminations or drugs, a "bed" baby. I ventured that the baby girl was making one last comeback, but Laurel thought otherwise. She told me that she had really bid her goodbye after Eric's birth and had planted an antique rose bush outside the bedroom window in her honor. Weeks later she phoned and said, "I must have done a pretty good job of letting go, because my amnio just revealed another baby boy. And Tabsh said he looked 'perfect.'"

Laurel's second pregnancy passed uneventfully except for back pain aggravated by osteoporosis and the care of a pre-schooler. The mild dose of steroids that Tabsh had prescribed kept the lupus at bay. Logan was delivered vaginally, a heroic feat due only to Laurel's fierce determination and Tabsh's remarkable skill.

Her lesson: "Sure, bad things can happen to good people,

but nothing stays bad forever. Hang in there and you'll be rewarded."

****

Another story that may inspire you is about my dearest Renee.

Thirty-three-year-old Renee had waded through twenty-one months of unexplained infertility. Her husband, Ken, had a King Kong sperm count—over two hundred million. Her laparoscopy, performed by a prominent infertility specialist, disclosed healthy insides, yet she couldn't get pregnant. She worried that since she had helped me research this book, she knew too much about the impediments to fertility and was mentally borrowing trouble.

She took Chlomid for six months and then graduated to Metrodin, all this time with accompanying inseminations and stress levels that rose accordingly. Desiring a second opinion, she journeyed to New York Hospital's Center for Reproductive Medicine and Infertility, which had boasted over the phone of a fifty percent pregnancy rate for their IVF program. (There isn't a clinic in any country, including this one, with a success rate that even approaches fifty percent.) "The place felt like a factory," she recalled. "I had to wait three hours and saw the doctor for five minutes. She never examined me and had no records from my California doctor."

Renee was sent to a nurse to schedule her IVF appointment. She had to accommodate her graduate school commitments because the procedure would require a two-week stay in New York. The center had promised to call her. They never did. She left ten messages. Renee finally gave up and arranged for the procedure at home in Los Angeles in two month's time.

To give her body a break, she'd gone off the fertility drugs. When she knew she was ovulating, she decided to take matters into her own hands. Surrounded by her crystals, her Woo-woo doll, and white light, Renee and Ken made love. He had tied a yellow bandanna at the base of his penis because he thought it would make him "shoot farther."

Immediately after they finished, her husband got teary-eyed, absolutely certain they had conceived. As you already know, she stood on her head for thirty minutes, with his help. They subsequently dreamed of babies. Three weeks later, she was pregnant.

"It's bad enough that your sex life becomes a chore during infertility," Renee confided, "but now I'm pregnant, we're scared to have sex." I remember being afraid to have an orgasm when I was carrying Mimi, worried that the uterine contractions would discharge the baby. I know most doctors tell you that it's safe to have orgasms, but many infertile couples who conceive don't want to tempt fate. Besides, it's been so long that they've had good sex that they feel they can wait a little longer.

Renee and her husband suffered three scares during their nine months. At six weeks, with Ken out of town, she awoke with pelvic pain on one side so intense that she called him in the middle of the night and talked to him for four hours until she could call her doctor in the morning. Renee felt hysterically frightened, fearing an ectopic pregnancy, but after her ultrasound, her doctor reassured her that the pain was caused by a leftover cyst from the Metrodin and not to worry.

When an AFP test, conducted at fourteen weeks, came back positive, indicating possible genetic defects, Renee recalls, "I flipped."

She later discovered that AFP tests are notorious for false-positive results. A nurse in her obstetrician's office informed her that out of every one hundred women with a positive result, ninety-eight are false. Even though she was only thirty-three, the AFP results required that she have an amnio. The doctor who performed her procedure said that the baby's neck looked "too fat, which was consistent with Down's syndrome." "But my husband and my father have thick necks. Could it be heredi-tary?" she asked. The doctor said no.

Also, he informed her that one chamber in the baby's heart seemed to be developing more slowly than the others, but told her not to worry because, "These things can fix themselves before birth." Thankfully, her amnio results two weeks later indicated that she was carrying a healthy baby boy.

Harrison arrived right on time, beautiful and whole, weigh-ing six pounds, eight ounces. He was the spitting image of his Daddy. He, too, possessed a gentle contentedness that seems characteristic of post-infertility babies. Maybe they just look that way through their worn-down parents' eyes, but I don't think so. I believe it's because they know how much they were wanted.

When Harrison was a little more than two, Renee and Ken knew they wanted another child. "It might take us a few years," they thought, "We'd better start trying now."

Two weeks later, Renee thought she had the flu. "I got pregnant the first time we tried," she told me.

During her amnio at seventeen weeks, the doctor told her she had another boy and he had a spot on his kidney. "It could be a million things, but most likely, it's nothing." he said. After two agonizing weeks of waiting, it *was* nothing.

After nine hours of labor, Renee delivered baby Marshall, weighing seven pounds, ten ounces. Harrison was potty trained within four weeks of his brother's birth.

Her lesson: "This might be hard to hear, but I believe babies come when they're supposed to and you get the one that's right for you. I was waiting for a baby, but Harrison was waiting for me to be ready."

****

Renee met a woman named Helene, who worked for Renee's father. She was also thirty-three, had been infertile for five years and had been on Chlomid for sixteen months. After she and Helene began commiserating by phone for a few months, Renee got pregnant.

She convinced Helene she could also help herself. She sent Helene a rose quartz crystal and told her to stand on her head. Helene conceived nine weeks later. She had a positive AFP fright like Renee, but all ended well and she is now the mother of a healthy two-and-a-half year old boy, Ryan. I've just learned that Ryan has a sibling on the way—another baby born of the bed.

****

Donna, a former New York colleague of Jim's, started her infertility saga with one fallopian tube and the news that her husband had no live sperm. They were advised to proceed with donor sperm. Another doctor saw evidence of some live sperm and urged them to try Pergonal and artificial inseminations. Her husband provided three ejaculations, which were distilled down to one good shot for each attempt they made.

After six grueling months, she got pregnant while I was carrying Mimi and delivered a healthy baby girl who looked exactly like her father.

Counting their blessings, Donna and her husband settled in and resumed their lives. We lost touch due to my divorce. Two years later, she appeared at Mimi's third birthday party with a tiny bundle in her arms. She had had another baby girl, this time conceived the old fashioned way. A few years later, I heard from Mimi that she had given birth to a third baby girl.

****

Bette was another friend of Renee's and mine, who had tried sporadically for nine years to get pregnant. Her periods were never regular, and she confessed that she'd always felt deep down that she'd never conceive. But she still she kept trying.

Her husband's sperm count was normal. Beginning when

she was thirty, they bounced from doctor to doctor. She had many cycles on Chlomid and Pergonal with inseminations that never worked. She would take off three months after each cycle to keep sane. At thirty-five, after three more diagnostic surgeries, one doctor decided to test her husband to see if his sperm could penetrate eggs. He failed the test. They were furious that it had taken five years to find that the problem wasn't hers.

"I felt the world was ending," she remembers. A varicocele was performed on her husband and soon after, he passed the egg penetration test. But there were billing discrepancies with the doctor, so they left him behind. Bette and her husband felt like their problems were solved and decided to take eighteen months to try at home.

They were unsuccessful on their own, so they found a new doctor who recommended intermittent cycles of Pergonal and inseminations. After a few months, he suggested a simultaneous GIFT and IVF procedure. She claims she had no expectations and enjoyed good spirits as she approached this next hurdle.

The doctor put four fertilized eggs in her tubes (GIFT) and three in her uterus (IVF). Shortly afterward, the spotting started. "I lost my mind," admits Bette. Then she got a positive blood test. "I was ecstatic. I told family and friends. For three hours, I thought I was pregnant." And then the doctor informed her that in fact, she was not. She had tested positive because of the many hormones she had taken prior to the procedure. This is what is called a "chemical pregnancy."

"I plummeted when I got the bad news," she acknowledges. "I thought it was my fault." Why? Because she and her husband had made love—no intercourse—but she'd had an orgasm. She feared that was the reason for the failure. (It wasn't.)

She wanted to quit, at least temporarily, but she couldn't, because at thirty-eight time was running out.

Three months later, Bette and her husband tried again. Since only three eggs were harvested and fertilized, IVF was the chosen route. Because of what had happened before, she wouldn't let her husband touch her.

Thirteen days later, Bette found out that she was pregnant. Her hormone levels were so high that twins were predicted. Two weeks later, the ultrasound revealed only one strong heartbeat.

"It was an enormously easy pregnancy," she remembers. Toward the end, her blood pressure elevated, so she began to anticipate an early delivery. I had more pelvic exams than anyone in history. They could never find a presenting part." (That meant the doctor couldn't feel the baby with his hands.) A C-section was scheduled and it proved fortuitous. Her baby was "traversed," or lying high across her belly. The umbilical cord was wrapped twice around its neck. The ultrasound never showed this perilous condition. But Bette, at thirty-nine, was finally rewarded. Spencer came into this world at six pounds, five ounces, looking exactly like his mother.

Her lesson: "Persevere. There is always a way to create your child. And if you can, take breaks in the process."

****

It is vital to remember that the stress of pregnancy after infertility is complex and chronic. After finally conceiving, both partners are often plagued by the dire possibilities that could jeopardize their baby's health. Of course, this situation is only intensified by a high-risk pregnancy.

One of the most remarkable survival stories I know of is that of Sam, the wife of one of Jim's colleagues. Her odyssey lasted over five years. With her first gynecologist, Sam took Chlomid for nine months. Then he referred her to a specialist who was performing various experimental techniques. For the next four months, he tried to pinpoint her problem.

"He drew blood every twenty minutes for five hours to see if my pituitary gland (which regulates ovulation) was working challenges taught me how to overcome my infertility. I am truly grateful for my disease. It has triggered all the important issues I needed to confront. It has brought me to my little girl and emboldened me to write this book. Those lessons still resonate today as I tackle each new challenge that my life presents. I have located inner resources I never knew existed. *Lesson #40: Out of something bad always comes something good.*

I always trust that I'm going to be okay. When I feel like I'm slipping, I trust I'll regain my footing. I still have some bad lupus days, albeit rarely, but even when I'm in the thick of it, I know it's going to end.

The lupus flares create a diversion from the actual stress that caused the original flare, because life, as I know it, literally stops when I have to concentrate on healing my body. For instance, if I'm hit with a bill I didn't expect, I may begin to worry how I'm going to pay it. If it's a huge amount, the worry might interrupt my sleep, which in turn will set off the lupus. At that point, I have to *let go* of the financial concern so I can sleep and restore my body. I have to trust that I will find a solution to the money problem, when I regain my strength. Answers are usually more likely to come when I am rested. And the lupus flares serve as reminders that I continually need to let go and trust that I will be okay. Besides, I know that without a healthy body I'm not going to be able to get around in this world. Not to mention that I have a little one who depends on me now.

So I don't fret anymore. I hit the bed for a day or two, surrender to the pain and plan for when I'm better. That way I don't waste my energy fighting it. If I've done all I can, I let it go. I trust that the best possible outcome will prevail. And it always does. Lupus provides me with a constant exercise in letting go. I never get rusty. *Lesson #41: When you have done all you can, surrender yourself to God.*

Along similar lines, Jack Kornfield, Ph.D., writes in his

article, "Seeing Our Problems as Blessings" (*New Age Journal*, October 1993):

> *Every life has periods and situations of great difficulty that call on our spirit. (We can) take our unwanted sufferings, the sorrows of our life and the struggles within us and...use them as a ground for nourishment of our patience and compassion, (as) the place to discover greater freedom.*

He offers this prayer:

> *Grant that I may be given appropriate difficulties and sufferings on this journey so that my heart may be truly awakened and my practice of liberation and universal compassion may be truly fulfilled.*

I agree with him when he says, "We can't always change the outside world, but we can change how we see it." His meditation which follows has helped me to investigate apparent misfortunes and find their hidden meanings and opportunities for personal growth.

Sit quietly and think of the difficulty that you face. Notice how it reflects in your body, mind, and heart. Begin to ask the following questions and listen inwardly for the answers:

1. How have I treated this difficulty so far?
2. How have I suffered by my own response and reaction to it?
3. What does this problem ask me to let go of?
4. What suffering is unavoidable, is my measure to keep?
5. What great lesson might it be able to teach me?
6. What is the...value hidden in this situation?

Kornfield explains that the understanding and changes of heart may come slowly. He advises repeating these reflections a number of times, listening each time for deeper answers from your body, mind and spirit.

Even though I had had my baby, I was left with some residual emotional pain. For a while, I felt guilty because I'd

broken through the infertility barrier. Why had I been rewarded when deserving others hadn't? On the other hand, I know the story of my journey inspired many people to carry on and ultimately triumph in their quest for children, so I wasn't the only one to benefit from my success.

When I wasn't feeling survivor guilt, I often felt like an ingrate. I felt uncomfortable complaining about the ordinary things that all new moms find difficult—no sleep, no sex, no energy, etc. It's common to overglorify parenting when you are infertile. But parenting an infant is exhausting and involves significant physical and psychological readjustments. My new problems were real. I had a premature infant and, regardless of what I'd been through, she had profound needs which I had to satisfy.

Having my baby didn't erase my infertility mindset, either. It's hard to shake years of intense longing and disappointment, especially if you've also had a tough pregnancy. Furthermore, I don't know if you ever totally recover from the trauma of infertility. It takes a long time to shift emotional gears and heal the scars, even though your crib may be full.

It's not that I was holding on to the pain. It's just that when trauma is severe, it can take years to recover. For example, many people in Los Angeles still feel the effects of the 1994 earthquake. Even though their houses have been bolstered and repaired, they were deeply shaken (figuratively and literally) where they slept and while they slept, in their most vulnerable places. They were swept up by the mysterious forces of nature, not unlike other mysterious forces of even greater magnitude that sweep souls onto this plane or prevent them from coming in. Some people may never feel totally safe again.

I consider myself a recovering infertility survivor. I still shudder when I glimpse back and allow myself to reexperience the ravaging pain from my years of infertility, it compounded by the disintegration of my third marriage. My relationship with

my family was fractured. I hadn't learned how to let go of the pain from my childhood. I wasn't *me* yet. I felt ragged and woeful and damaged and miserable. Infertility was the final blow. The lupus is what revived me. And therapy became my lifeline. Even now, the memory of those times before my enlightenment, hurts me to contemplate. I was in pieces then, not whole. Mimi may be eight-and-a-half, but I still have a visceral memory of my empty arms, my breaking heart, and my lonely life.

****

I marveled at Mimi every time she suckled my breasts. I couldn't believe that she had grown inside me and I was now feeding her with my body. I felt overjoyed that she was real and that we belonged to each other. In the beginning, I'd have dreams that I'd lost her or left her somewhere and I'd wake up and run in her room. I checked her often to make sure she was breathing. I still go into her room some nights just to gaze at her, incredulous that she is here, overwhelmed by the miracle of her life.

She is my joy, my heart, and thanks to Jim, the best thing I've ever done. We both feel so utterly blessed by her. I love my Mimi more than anything in the world; I never expected to feel this way about anyone. I'd throw myself in front of a bus for her. I would willingly die so she could live. So would her Daddy.

A child brings the divine gift of unconditional love into your life. And being a parent means you get to be a child all over again. With so many of us coming from variously dysfunctional families, having your own child is a chance for renewal and self-love at last. Nursing a little one is a great and lifelong exercise in spiritual resolution.

I'm sure you'll understand why I am convinced that miracles happen to people who believe in them. I have a very special child that is the product of my faith, hope, will, and love. I am

now emotionally and spiritually healthier than ever before. So what if I have lupus? I have peace in my soul. I feel safe and secure. I have the ability to see and know things. I have the ability to touch others wherever I go. The love I give returns to me tenfold. I am surrounded by loving people whom I respect and who respect me. I have my spiritual guides. I have love all around me. My dream, my child, is alive.

When I was a teenager and well into my twenties, I used to dream about being crowned Miss America, marrying Prince Charming, or receiving an Oscar. (Oh, to have such adulation and validation! And wouldn't that show all who'd sarcastically called me Sarah Bernhardt just how wrong they were?) Years ago, those were my escapes from whatever injustice or malady I was suffering at the moment. I also wanted a quick fix. Alcohol provided relief for a while, but as the highs became higher, the lows became increasingly more intense. Fortunately, my desire to have a child outweighed my need to obliterate my reality. I ceased my destructive behavior and said farewell to Cinderella, Snow White, Sleeping Beauty, and the Brass Ring. I no longer needed a Prince on a white horse. I'm riding my own horse, and I've been ennobled by my experiences.

Remember that initially I approached my infertility in my typical frenetic way, craving instant gratification and a fairy-tale ending. Had I become pregnant before learning all that I've shared with you, I wouldn't and couldn't have become the parent I am today. And any child I might have had would have paid the price of my ignorance. If your baby hasn't come yet, it may be because there is something you need to learn or do before its arrival. You just have to figure out what it is. It could really be that simple.

I want you to learn from my experience: you are never really stuck, you always have choices and options, and remember that no one can take your power away from you. I know

that no matter what happens, I'll be okay. You, too, can take care of yourself in any situation. By believing in your powers and present abilities, you can create a better future for yourself.

Most important, I know that at all times I am doing the best I can, and that's all any one of us, including you, can do. I finally let go of my Superwoman fantasies. What a relief to find the real me instead!

****

As I mentioned earlier, the lupus brought my marital woes to a fevered pitch. Since stress triggered the illness, the worse the stress got, the sicker I became. The sicker I got, the more unhappy Jim and I became. We were both completely unavailable for each other and the distance between us grew unbearable. So did the tension, and arguments and alienation ruled our lives. I worried how the turmoil would affect our baby's development.

I remember breastfeeding Mimi when she was close to a year old. I was rocking her in her room. Jim came in and a particularly nasty discourse ensued. The baby fussed because she knew from the volume of our dialogue and my body tension that we were fighting.

As Jim stormed out, I silently vowed to leave as soon as I felt physically able. Jim and I had both been raised in volatile households. I wanted a different life for my daughter and for me.

After almost eighteen months of therapy with Jim, I decided to leave him. I was thirty-eight years old with a broken-down body, and a nineteen-month-old angel, and I hadn't worked in five years. (Not to mention that this would be my third divorce. But I didn't let the numbers deter me.) I knew if I were ever to feel well again, I had to go. The stress of our failing marriage fueled the lupus and suffocated my spirit. I still loved Jim, but I recognized that our marriage would never

work. And so, with the help of all the women I hold dear, I found a small house to rent, took half of Jim's and my savings, scooped up my baby, and walked out.

The next few months took a toll on both of us, as we hammered out a divorce settlement with the lawyers. But once the legal documents were finalized, we began forging a friendship. We did this with care. We knew that we were going to be in each other's lives forever because we had a daughter to raise. I remember those first weekends when Jim would come to pick up Mimi for visits. Until that time, I had never been separated from her and I felt like my heart was being clenched by a big fist. She wasn't even potty-trained.

Jim's obvious devotion to Mimi allowed me to finally relax and accept the separations from her. Although he was dragged kicking and screaming into fatherhood, Jim has evolved into a fantastically attentive and compassionate parent. His life has been so positively transformed by Mimi that, despite our divorce, I feel everything has truly worked out for the best.

I see the way he looks at her and the emotions surge within me. There was a time when I longed for one of those looks. Now I'm grateful that she's getting them. Jim makes as much time for her as he can, given his busy traveling schedule. She accompanies him whenever she can and has visited more foreign countries than I'll ever see. On her first day in kindergarten, she stood up and talked about her three-week trip to Greece that summer.

I've never regretted my decision because I felt we had done everything we could to make the marriage work. Mimi is now a loving, shining third grader, with a delicious sense of humor and emotional maturity beyond her years. She is my heart. (I have just realized that I am going to be almost fifty when she starts junior high!) And while she's pretty well adjusted to our divorce, I doubt that her wish for our reconciliation, even though she lacks a conscious memory of us together, will ever die.

Fortunately for all three of us, Jim and I have managed to develop a new relationship based on respect, friendship and shared parenting duties. And sometimes when I have Mimi news, only his ear will do—he's the only person on the planet that's as captivated by her as I am. We depend on and support each other and feel mutual delight that we have all come so far.

Jim has enjoyed enormous success in the entertainment business and I have found my second passion in life after motherhood: my writing.

The lupus is well-controlled and my body becomes healthier with each passing year. (So much for this being a progressive disease.) I recently underwent an appendectomy and the removal of a tubal abscess (cause unknown), and received further confirmation of my miracle, eight years after the fact. My surgeon echoed Dr. Tabsh's words and amazement when he said, "I don't know how you ever got pregnant!"

My poor baby dog Alex, however, has entered the twilight of his life. As of this writing, at almost eleven, he has great difficulty walking, due to a degenerative nerve and bone condition. New, revolutionary medicine has staved off the inevitable, but it is with great sadness that Mimi and I watch him fail a little more each day, knowing we will ultimately have to decide when to let him go.

After a long separation from my parents and some of my brothers, I found forgiveness in my heart and we reconciled. Mimi inherited a huge, extended family. I bought my own home after the divorce and have never felt more satisfied or content than I do today.

I never expected to be dating in my forties, and initially I worried about my "marketability," with a toddler and a chronic illness, until a male friend set me straight. "Mimi and the lupus are great screening devices," he reassured me. He proved to be right.

It's been a trip. By the way, those stories you hear about the

surge in a woman's libido at forty, are true. Something to look forward to!

And though I never imagined myself in my present circumstances, life happily goes on. *Lesson #42: You don't always get what you want, but you always get what you need.*

To stay on the right track, according to Joseph Campbell, "Follow your bliss."

Here's how I keep it together, and I invite you to consider any of the following realizations as guidelines for your own path.

Katie's Eleven Commandments

I try always to remember that life is a journey, not a destination, and to listen to the quiet sounds along the way.

I trust myself and my judgement, because I really do know what's best for me. I don't worry about trusting others because I'll know instinctively if I can or can't.

I will never again allow anyone to mistreat me because now I have the tools to protect myself in any situation.

I take care of myself and am true to myself before all others and I expect others to be able to care for themselves. If they cannot, I accept that I cannot fix them and I will detach in the most loving way possible.

I am dedicated to being honest with myself and others at all costs.

I remind myself that I am a good mother, and as a good mother, I must take good care of myself or I will be no good to my child.

I respect and love my body just the way it is and I care for it lovingly.

I realize that when I take care of myself, the universe takes care of me.

I love myself, for what I am today, not for what I am going to be tomorrow. I forgive myself for past mistakes and I let them go.

I am worthy of all good things, I am entitled to miracles and I deserve every wonderful wind that blows my way.

And I know my future is glowing and bright, because I have the love of God and that of my friends and family to support me. And best of all, I have myself.

Good luck, Godspeed and much love!

Dear Reader,

When you get pregnant, please write to me and share your success. I would like to hear your story—what you did, and what worked for you.
    Good luck!

Love,

Katie

Katie Boland
c/o Underwood Books
PO Box 1609
Grass Valley, CA 95945

RESOURCE GUIDE

READING LIST

HEALING MIND, HEALTHY WOMAN
by Alice D. Domar, Ph.D.
Henry Holt 1996

LOVE, MEDICINE & MIRACLES
Lessons Learned About Self-Healing From a Surgeon's Experience with Exceptional Patients
by Bernie S. Siegel, M.D.
HarperCollins 1990

ANATOMY OF AN ILLNESS AS PERCEIVED BY THE PATIENT
Reflections on Healing and Regeneration
by Norman Cousins
Bantam Books 1985

YOU CAN HEAL YOUR LIFE
by Louise L. Hay
Hay House, Inc. 1987

PEACE, LOVE & HEALING
Bodymind Communication & the Path to Self-Healing: An Exploration
by Bernie S. Siegel, M.D.
HarperCollins 1989

GETTING PREGNANT WHEN YOU THOUGHT YOU COULDN'T
The Interactive Guide That Helps You Up the Odds
by Helene S. Rosenberg, Ph.D. and Yakov M. Epstein, Ph.D.
Warner Books 1993

THE FERTILITY SOLUTION
A Revolutionary Approach to Reversing Infertility
by A. Toth, M.D.
Atlantic Monthly Press 1991

MEDITATIONS

Creative Visualization and Meditation Exercises to Enrich Your Life
by Shakti Gawain
New World Library 1991

MINDING THE BODY, MENDING THE MIND
by Joan Borysenko, Ph.D.
Bantam 1987

A RETURN TO LOVE
Reflections on the Principles of "A COURSE IN MIRACLES"
by Marianne Williamson
HarperCollins 1992

HEAD FIRST
The Biology of Hope
by Norman Cousins
Dutton 1989

BRAIN LONGEVITY
by Dharma Singh Khalsa, M.D.
Warner Books 1997

KUNDALINI YOGA
The Flow of Eternal Power
by Shakti Parwha Kaur Khalsa
Time Capsule Books 1996

OPTIMUM HEALTH
A Natural Lifesaving Prescription for Your Body and Mind
by Stephen Sinatra, M.D.
Bantam Books 1996

HEALING AND THE MIND
by Bill Moyers
Doubleday 1993

COMPLETE AROMATHERAPY HANDBOOK
Essential Oils for Radiant Health
by Susanne Fischer-Rizzi

SEX FOR ONE
The Joy of Selfloving
by Betty Dodson, Ph.,D.
Three Rivers Press 1996

THE EROTIC ADVENTURES OF
SLEEPING BEAUTY
by Anne Rice writing as A.N. Roquelaure
Penguin Books 1985

HEALING WORDS
The Power of Prayer and the Practice of Medicine
by Larry Dossey, M.D.
Harper San Francisco 1993

OUT OF THE DARKNESS INTO
THE LIGHT
by Gerald Jampolsky, M.D.
Bantam Books 1989

THE WELLNESS BOOK
by Herbert Benson, M.D.
Fireside/Simon and Schuster 1993

INTERIOR DESIGN WITH
FENG SHUI
by Sarah Rossbach
Arkana/Penguin Books 1991

THE CONCEPTION MANDALA
Creative Techniques for Inviting a Child into Your Life
by Mark Olsen and Samuel Avital
Destiny Books 1992

CONSCIOUS CONCEPTION
by Jeannine Parvati Baker and
Frederick Baker
Firestone Publishing and North
Atlantic Books 1986

ADOPTION WISDOM
by Marlou Russell, Ph.D.
Broken Branch Productions 1996

A WOMAN'S BOOK OF LIFE
by Joan Borysenko, Ph.D.
Riverhead Books 1996

WORDS THAT HEAL
by Douglas Bloch
Bantam Books 1990

ALTERNATIVE THERAPIES
& PRACTIONERS

International Kundalini Yoga Teachers'
Association
(505) 753-0423

Sat Jivan Kaur Khalsa
Kundalini Yoga Fertility Instructor
(212) 995-0571

International Chiropractors' Association Council on Chiropractic Pediatrics
(703) 528-5000

Christine Anderson, D.C., D.I.C.C.P.
Board certified chiropractor treating
infertility
6565 Sunset Blvd, Suite 302
Los Angeles, CA 90028
(213) 467-6348

American Association of Acupuncture
and Oriental Medicine
433 Front Street
Catasauqua, PA 18032
(610) 266-1433

Daoshing Ni, L.Ac., D.O.M., Ph.D.
Infertility specialist
Union of Tao and Man Traditional
Acupuncture Inc.
1314 Second Street, Suite 101
Santa Monica, CA 90401
(310) 917-2267

L.Lou Paget, Sex educator
The Sexuality Seminars
(310) 556-3623

Good Vibrations Catalogue
(800) 289-8423
Billy Blanks World Training Center
(818) 906-8528

Marie Garcia
Feng Shui consultant
(909) 599-2598

SUPPORT GROUPS

RESOLVE, Inc.
National Headquarters
1310 Broadway
Somerville, MA 02144
(617) 623-1156
Helpline: (617) 623-0744

American Society of Reproductive
Medicine
(formerly the American Fertility Society)
1209 Montgomery Highway
Birmingham, AL 35216-2809
(205) 978-5000

The National Committee on Adoption
1930 17th Street NW
Washington, D.C. 20009
(202) 328-1200

A.M.E.N.D.
Provides one-on-one support for parents coping with miscarriage, stillbirth or the loss of newborn infants
4324 Berrywick Terrace
St. Louis, MO 63128
(314) 487-7528

SHARE
Pregnancy and Infant Loss Support, Inc.
St. Joseph's Health Center
300 First Capitol Drive
St. Charles, MO 63301
(314) 947-6164
Offers referrals to support groups nationwide

MIND/BODY PROGRAMS FOR INFERTILITY

The Mind/Body Medical Institute
Deaconess Hospital
One Deaconess Road
Boston, MA 02215
(617) 632-9525
(for tapes also)

Morristown Memorial Hospital
95 Mt. Kemble Avenue
Morristown, NJ 07962
(201) 971-4575

Riverside Methodist Hospital
3535 Olentangy River Road
Columbus, OH 43214
(614) 566-4050

Memorial Hospital Southwest
7500 Beechnut, Suite 321
Houston, TX 77074
(713) 776-5020

St. Peter's Medical Center
254 Easton Avenue
New Brunswick, NJ 08901
(908) 745-8528

NOTES

Chapter II: Psyched Out

1. D. S. Khalsa and C. Stauth, *Brain Longevity*, Warner Books, (1997): 115-122

2. Ibid

3. Ibid

4. F. Facchinetti, K. Demyttenaere, L. Fioroni, I. Neri and A. Genazzani "Psychosomatic disorders related to gynecology." *Psychotherapy Psychosomatic* 58 (1992): 137-154

5. M.B. Rosenthal, "Infertility: psychotherapeutic issues" *Treating Diverse Disorders with Psychotherapy* (1991): 61-71

6. F. Facchinetti, K. Demyttenaere, L. Fioroni, I. Neri and A. Genazzani "Psychosomatic disorders related to gynecology." *Psychotherapy Psychosomatic* 58 (1992): 137-154

7. N. Benazon, J. Wright, and S. Sabourin. "Stress, sexual satisfaction and marital adjustment in infertile couples." *Journal of Sex & Marital Therapy* 18(4) (1992): 273-284

8. S.H. McDaniel, J, Hepworth, and W. Doherty. "Medical family therapy with couples facing infertility." *The American Journal of Family Therapy* 20 (2) (1992) 101-120

9. F. Facchinette, K. Demyttenaere, L. Fioroni, I. Beri and A. Genazzani. "Psychosomatic disorders related to gynecology." *Psychotherapy Psychosomatic* 58 (1992): 137-154

10. A.D. Domar, *Healing Mind, Healthy Women*, Henry Holt (1996): 229-65

11. Ibid 237

12. Ibid 238

13. Ibid 259

Chapter VI: Live Acts

1. F. Facchinette, K. Demyttenaere, L. Fioroni, I. Beri and A. Genazzani. "Psychosomatic disorders related to gynecology." *Psychotherapy Psychosomatic* 58 (1992): 137-154.

2. S. McDaniel, J. Hepworth and W. Doherty. "Medical family therapy with couples facing infertility." *The American Journal of Family Therapy* 20 (2) (1992): 101-120

3. Ibid.

4. M. Rosenthal, "Infertility: psychotherapeutic issues." *Treating Diverse Disorders with Psychotherapy* 58 (1991): 61-71.

5. Ibid.

INDEX